Coping
with Prednisone*

(*and Other Cortisone-Related Medicines)

Coping with Prednisone*

(*and Other Cortisone-Related Medicines)

It may work miracles, but how do you handle the side effects?

Eugenia Zukerman

and Julie R. Ingelfinger, M.D.

St. Martin's Press ⁂ New York

Design by Jenny Dossin

Library of Congress Cataloging-in-Publication Data

Zukerman, Eugenia.
    Coping with prednisone*: (*and other cortisone-related medicines)
    Eugenia Zukerman and Julie R. Ingelfinger. —1st ed.
        p.   cm.
    Includes bibliographical references.
    ISBN 0-312-15502-6
    1. Prednisone—Side effects.   2. Glucocorticoids—Side effects.
    I. Ingelfinger, Julie R.   II. Title
    RM292.4P7Z   1997
    615' .364—dc21   97-6062
                                                          CIP

First Edition: September 1997

10 9 8 7 6 5 4 3 2 1

This book is dedicated to
Stanley R. Rich
our father
in loving memory

Acknowledgments

Many of our friends and family members provided invaluable advice by talking with us, reading drafts, and suggesting additional topics about steroids. We would especially like to thank our literary agent, Loretta Barrett, whose help and suggestions encouraged us to do this project; our editor, Hope Dellon, who provided clarifying insights and stylistic pointers; and Julie's son, Franz Ingelfinger, who verified information for the appendix.

Table of Contents

Coping with Prednisone: Who Needs This Book?

An estimated one million people in the United States take high doses of prednisone and related drugs (glucocorticoids) yearly. Cortisone was first available in the early 1950s and was touted as a wonder drug for its miraculous effectiveness in alleviating a wide range of serious illnesses and conditions. Although its side effects were simultaneously apparent, its benefits seemed by far to outweigh its risks. There is at present no preparation of this medication that totally prevents the adverse effects of the drug. Many doctors neither communicate the potential magnitude of the side effects nor understand how profoundly these effects may upset their patients. Strategies for dealing with taking this potent medication are too rarely offered.

Coping with Prednisone is for those one million individuals per year who will be on sustained courses of high-dose steroids. It is also for their significant others and/or caregivers, and it is for doctors and health-care workers and for anyone else who is interested in wellness.

Eugenia I am a flutist with an international career; I am also a television correspondent and a writer. My schedule requires nonstop work and megawatt energy, and never in a thousand years did I imagine that I could be felled by—of all things—a rare lung disease. But there I was in a hospital, breathless, weak, being told that unless I took high doses of prednisone, my disease could kill me. I didn't want to die; I obviously had to take those massive doses. But I also knew that prednisone could distort my face and body, and I had to worry about going on television and stepping onto a stage. I knew it had other side effects that could further compromise my work. My multiple livelihoods were at stake. The first lung specialist to whom I had been sent wanted to cure my disease. He did not, however, seem very worried about the possible side effects the necessary medication might cause. This book came about because of the counsel and compassion I received from my sister, Julie R. Ingelfinger, M.D. Her help, advice, and support throughout the more than ten months of my treatment with prednisone was invaluable to me and, it turns out, to her, too. We decided to write this book together, in hopes that our experience will be a guide to others who are coping with prednisone.

Julie   I have been a physician for over twenty-five years and work at Massachusetts General Hospital, a major teaching hospital of Harvard Medical School, where I am happily involved in patient care, teaching, and basic research. In my work as a pediatric nephrologist (kidney specialist for children) I have often needed to prescribe large doses of corticosteroids to treat specific kidney problems in children, and so I felt that I was aware of their many benefits as well as their side effects. In fact, in order to be helpful to my patients and their parents, I had long maintained a list of steroid side effects that I distributed whenever I needed to give a patient steroids for a sustained period of time. I have to confess that I felt pleased with this list and my prescribing habits until my sister Eugenia was told that she had to take high-dose steroids for at least several months. Her alarm and dismay seemed understandable, but I don't think I really "got" how tough it is for even the most motivated patient to be on this kind of medication until it hit so close to home. Both Eugenia and I were struck by how little information is available for a patient in this situation, and so we decided to use the experience we had during Eugenia's treatment—as sisters, as doctor and patient, and as people who want to help others—to put together a primer on steroids for people who need high doses for a long period of time.

Accordingly, this book is for patients who are on (or are going to be on) oral steroids for more than a two-week period, at a dose far greater than that produced by the body's own adrenals (typically, at a dose of prednisone—a form of glucocorticoid most commonly prescribed at or exceeding 0.25 milligram per kilogram of body weight per day). Thus it is not a book for people taking a five-day course of prednisone for poison ivy or for those who use over-the-counter steroid cream for an itch or a bug bite.

Our hope is that this book can help those needing long-term steroids to understand what steroids do, why they are prescribed, what the side effects are, and how these side effects can be minimized.

Terms Used in This Book

Many patients say they are "on cortisone" or "on steroids" or "on prednisone" when they are taking any kind of glucocorticoid. Formally, all of the medications we discuss in this book are *glucocorticoids,* substances produced or related to those produced in the adrenal glands. Many terms are used interchangeably to describe these medications. Here is the list of how we will use these terms:

Steroids: glucocorticoids, corticosteroids
Prednisone: the most commonly prescribed glucocorticoid

The names of other glucocorticoids are found in tables in the appendix. However, we will generally use the terms *steroids* or *prednisone.*

Don't confuse the use of the term steroids *in this book with anabolic steroids, often abused by athletes and bodybuilders as "performance enhancers." Anabolic steroids are a different type of steroid and not considered here.*

How
Bloated
Will I Be?

Eugenia "You are one sick puppy," the doctor tells me as he looks at the x-rays that have just been taken. Having consulted various doctors who could find nothing wrong with me, I had finally been sent to a lung specialist, and bingo, he found the problem. But now I begin to panic. What is it? A tumor? Cancer? But the doctor instantly adds, "The good news is—this can be treated."

I'm sick but treatable! Life is good!

After six months of feeling ill and exhausted, during which I had repeated bouts of bronchitis, odd spiky fevers, a chronic cough, there was finally a definitive diagnosis—eosinophilic pneumonitis, a disease that is neither viral nor bacterial in origin, the cause of which is elusive but results in massive inflammation that severely affects the ability of the lungs to oxygenate blood.

"It's very rare," I am told, with a smile. Now like a praised, if sick, puppy, I waggle with a weird sense of pride. Of course I have a rare disease! And rare it looks on the illuminated x-ray, all those white clouds floating around in my chest cavity, called, I am told, pulmonary infiltrates.

Suddenly I feel infiltrated, invaded. Violated. Something has triggered a massive allergic attack in my body, and the eosinophilic blood cells have responded by marching into my lungs and taking over. No wonder I've had trouble breathing.

A professional flute player who toots around the world, I turned fifty at about the same time my pulmonary problem kicked in. Concerts became a challenge. Sustaining long phrases made me feel as if I were drowning. I muddled through and went to various doctors, but none heard anything serious through a stethoscope. I was left thinking, *I'm fifty. This is how it feels.*

But now I am redeemed. I have been x-rayed and diagnosed, and my problem is treatable. "And the medication is . . . ?" I ask, eager for a quick fix.

My doctor looks serious. A pause, then, "Prednisone."

"Prednisone," I repeat, thinking instantly of my close friend, the cellist Jacqueline du Pre, who took prednisone for her multiple sclerosis, causing her angelic face to puff up and splotch and her body to spread. But Jacky was on massive doses, and surely I wouldn't have to be. "How much prednisone?" I ask.

My doctor looks even more serious. "Sixty milligrams a day of prednisone, at first."

"Sixty!? At first?" I gulp. "What are we talking about here?"

More serious yet: "Long-term therapy."

"How long?"

"Possibly six months. Probably longer."

My brain sizzles. "So are you saying I'll be on massive doses for almost a year?"

"The doses will be reduced, slowly," he says, "but the eosinophils must be suppressed, and stay suppressed, or you run the risk of having the infiltrates return. . . ."

Now I really panic. Then I tell myself to stay calm. After all, there's good news here. Not only do I finally know what's going on, but it's treatable. Yet the panic returns as I realize I have to look presentable, on the stage and on television. I know that prednisone can make you bloated and distort your features. For fifteen years I have been the arts correspondent for CBS News's "Sunday Morning." And there's still a double standard—male TV personalities can look plump and rumpled; women on TV are expected to look slim and sleek.

"Will I blow up?" I ask.

The doctor waits a beat before pronouncing a definitive, "Yes."

"It's my face! It's my body!" I blurt. "I won't take that much prednisone. I'd rather die!" Overdramatic, I know, and narcissistic as hell, but, hey, I'm fifty and it's bad enough feeling vulnerable physically but professionally too?

The doctor's face registers bemused concern. "You will take the prednisone," he says, "or you *could* die."

That shuts me up. Death or distortion? No contest. I mumble a contrite, "OK," then ask, just in case, "But isn't there some other drug I could take?"

"I'm afraid not."

I nod and swallow hard. I will blow up. I'm going to look awful. I will have to wear a paper bag over my head for six months or more. I will take a leave of absence from life. Become a recluse. Hide in my room. Or, I realize with a flash of hope, I can call my big sister.

Julie Rich Ingelfinger, M.D., is the head of the Pediatric Nephrology Unit at Massachusetts General Hospital in Boston and an Associate Professor at Harvard Medical School. She was in *Boston Magazine*'s listing of the best doctors in town. She's a top-of-the-line medical maven and knows her stuff and will save me from the side effects of prednisone. Two and a half years older than I, my sister has always been my greatest ally, except of course for the time when I was two and she cut off all my hair. Our mom and dad apparently found her sitting on the floor holding my curls saying, "It will grow back; it will grow back. . . ."

Our sibling rivalry stopped some fifteen years after the scissors incident, and we've been the best of friends ever since. I call her up at the hospital, where she is putting in long weeks, directing her unit and her busy research lab, and add my lungs and their care to her already heavy burden. But Best Big Sister in the World that she is, she swings into action, contacting my doctor in New York, arranging for my x-rays and CAT scans to be sent up to Boston for consultations. She wants to check on the diagnosis, make sure all possible tests have been done. Meanwhile, she says, I have to bite the bullet and take the damned prednisone.

"But, Julie," I protest, "my doctor says I'll blow up. My career is over!"

"Don't be stupid," she says. "You can still play concerts and be on air looking a bit plump. But there *are* things you can do to prevent the bloat."

I knew she'd come through! "Such as?"

"Exercise. Diet. For starters, no salt, no sugar, no simple carbos, and I'll figure out the rest," she says, with complete confidence. "I'll ask my colleagues. Don't worry. We'll beat the prednisone problems."

Yay, team! I think. But I'm still worried. I can't help it: I'm the one who could end up looking like Moby Dick.

2

Aren't
Wet Feet Petty
at a Time
Like This?

Julie   My sister Genie, Eugenia to her friends in adult-hood but Genie to me, once acted surprised when I ran to help someone having convulsions on the T (the Metropolitan Transit Authority Boston subway system of *Charlie* "oh, he never returned" fame) while we were going somewhere with our young children. "What are you doing?" she screeched at me.

"I'm a doctor!" I yelled back.

Later she said, "You know, I completely forgot that you're a doctor." But years have gone by, and mostly she doesn't forget this. Like many doctors, I sometimes would rather be a regular family member, not a doctor who is also a sister, daughter, mother, et cetera. It works in funny ways.

So, when my sister Genie called upset about a scary and serious pulmonary illness and its recommended treatment—high-dose glucocorticoids—I felt like her sister, not like a doctor. I was upset, too. It was ironic, my flutist sister having a lung problem! How unfair, how potentially devastating! Then, as physicians often do when they or family members have a medical problem, I "white-coated." I quickly remembered I was the doctor/sister, and my upset merged into wanting to solve everything—to be sure that Genie's diagnosis was correct and that the treatment recommended was "the best." I thought, *I am no expert in pulmonary problems, but as a kidney specialist I do very often prescribe steroids—cortisone, prednisone, prednisolone, et cetera—as these agents have multiple roles in treating kidney diseases, so I can help.*

The type of steroids prescribed to treat my sister's problem, eosinophilic pneumonitis, is in the class of steroids called glucocorticoids, potent medications that, while very effective in the treatment of a myriad of ailments, have a lot of serious side effects. Like most doctors, I focus on curing disease. I consider the side effects, but I don't dwell on them, especially if the illness is serious and the therapy can control or cure it.

Like most patients, Eugenia wanted to be well, but she was utterly aghast at the thought of side effects, especially visible ones. So, when she asked me about what to do to prevent side effects from high-dose steroids, I had multiple reactions. One was to remember a colleague who runs a dialysis unit and posts on his wall an old *New Yorker* cartoon, which shows Moses talking to a bunch of sandal-wearing people in long garments, shepherds' staffs in their hands, crossing a body of water parted in front of them, saying, "Look, Aaron, don't you think complaining about wet feet is petty at a time like this?" Still, with my doctor hat on, I could truthfully say, "I always try to tell my patients about the side effects of the medicines that I prescribe, so of course I have information for you."

After all, for glucocorticoids I actually already had in hand an "information sheet" for kidney patients. But when I looked at it, it was just one page. I know my sister—she'd need more than this to satisfy her. It also made me wonder—how did *my* patients feel? Maybe they, too, needed more than one page. So, as Genie and I talked, I thought about the kind of things my colleagues and I recommend to patients we put on steroids who want to avoid weight gain and redistribution:

AVOID SALT

AVOID SIMPLE CARBOHYDRATES

KEEP CALORIES DOWN

I have convenient no-added-salt diets and "foods to avoid" and "foods to use." But none of these lists gives any information about how effective they will be or about how anyone came up with these bits of advice in the first place. I had pieced together information and advice culled from colleagues and patients. It hardly represented hard data. I decided to look in the National Library of Medicine files by doing computer searches on "BRS Colleague" and "Paperchase" back to 1966, to see if anyone had written about the basis behind the recommended way to avoid weight gain and weight redistribution while on steroids. I found almost nothing about this aspect of glucocorticoid usage. Certainly nothing to back up my supposedly practical recommendations. And nothing to support the patient. I called about ten colleagues, all of whom, like me, are medical academics who prescribe a lot of steroids. Nobody knew any more than I did. Nobody had any real information. We docs had *tons* of information about the anti-inflammatory effects of glucocorticoids, about how glucocorticoids interact with genes, with lymphocytes, with other hormones. We knew how these agents worked to control disease, but we didn't know much about their side effects in the weight gain department. Every treatise published about steroids describes the redistribution of body fat stores and weight gain seen in steroid excess, yet none explains exactly *why* patients on glucocorticoids gain and redistribute weight. And none tells patients or health-care professionals how to cope with this! And that was only the beginning: Steroids have a lot of other side effects. *What about those?* I wondered.

I decided that my colleagues and I have been unintentionally glib. By virtue of focusing on illness and how to cure or control it, we have neglected some aspects of therapy important to patients and their families—and, indeed, to us doctors when we ourselves are on medicine—what does the treatment do to the quality of life? The more Genie and I talked, the more we felt we should make an attempt to deal with the ignorance about weight gain and other steroid side effects. So we decided to write this handbook about how to handle being on glucocorticoids.

3

They've
Kicked In

Eugenia I can breathe! In less than twenty-four hours I am practicing the flute with the kind of breath control I've been missing for months. And all it took was one day and sixty milligrams of prednisone! I will be on this megadose for an unspecified amount of time, until the X rays are clear, and I seem to be, as the doctor puts it, "doing better." I feel a little shaky, and weird, but I can play the flute! I'm not just doing better. I'm doing fine!

But now it's three days later. The middle of the night. I'm squinting into the mirror in the bathroom. Only seventy-two hours into my prednisone therapy and my face is definitely spreading. I'm already turning into a pumpkin. I look again, closer. I study my face. Where are those vertical lines above my top lip and the parentheses on either side of my mouth? They're gone! Could this mean that as I puff up I'll wrinkle down? Nice trade-off. I stare at myself, troubled nonetheless. I go back to bed. I can't sleep. I lie there, tossing and turning, and, one hour later, I get up to look in that funhouse mirror again. This time I put on my glasses, without which, I remember, I am legally blind. Now I see plenty of wrinkles around my mouth. *Thank God for wrinkles,* I think. I'll take haghood over puffdom any day, I decide, and go back to sleep.

The next morning a fax arrives from Julie—her information sheet titled "Effects of Glucocorticoids during Ongoing Therapy." My own doctor here in New York had suggested that I *not* read the "adverse reactions" list that accompanied my large bottle of prednisone. Paternalistic and pandering though his advice may have been, I did not question him further. Instead, I requested information from Julie, which she quickly sent. But as I read the faxed page, I felt more and more nauseated. I was informed that my medication could cause "cushingoid features"—basically, a fat, flushed face and weight gain around the trunk of the body, sometimes on the upper back and chest, acne, increase in body hair, thin and fragile skin, stretch marks. The immune system is compromised; not only might moods swing, but the patient could become psychotic and get ulcers and cataracts and pseudo brain tumors, and . . .

My head spins. Maybe I'll be able to breathe, but I'll have pimples and hair on my chest, and my mind will bend, my eyes will fuzz, and probably I'll go stark raving mad! Needing reassurance, I try to reach Julie, but she's unavailable. In a state of turmoil I march off to my daily visit to the doctor and announce, "I've read about the side effects of prednisone. It's my body, and I'm not putting anything this poisonous into it. There's got to be something else I can take."

"There isn't," he says.

"There isn't," Julie corroborates, when I reach her by phone later on. "Try to be reasonable. Get a grip!"

I do. I try to reason with myself. I must focus on getting well, on being able to play the flute. I must stop worrying about side effects. I attempt to shape up. I even try to rest. I cancel a month of concerts, doctor's orders. It's ironic that the most enjoyable activity—making music—is also the most stressful. Travel is exhausting. Stepping out onstage is high-risk. It takes a lot of nervous energy. And I need to lie low until I'm stronger. But I can still do some of my CBS work. I tell a pal, a cameraman at CBS, about my condition and the medication I have to take.

"I shot a 'piece' about the doctor who invented cortisone," he tells me. "He was honored for discovering this wonder drug, but then when his patients started getting all the nasty side effects, he committed suicide."

Thank you for sharing, I thought. But I am not about to put a bullet through my head. I'm going to beat the blues and the bloat. I'm on a rigid no-salt, no-sugar, low-starch diet, and I don't feel the least bit deprived, for this reason—what I eat is the one thing I can control about my body right now. I do, however, already have some annoying side effects:

1) *An overgrowth of yeast in my mouth, or thrush, sometimes associated with high doses of prednisone.* My tongue and the roof of my mouth and my throat are coated with a nasty white yeasty overgrowth. The antidote, prescribed by my doctor—I gargle four times a day with a disgusting potion of liquid nystatin and spit it out. And I also brush my tongue with hydrogen peroxide, something also suggested by my doctor. And, because it seems logical, I am eating no yeast products whatsoever—no bread, no packaged rice and other products that have yeast in the labels. The combination of nystatin, peroxide, and no yeast seems to be working. In a few days, the thrush begins to vanish.

2) *Major munchies. My appetite is out of control.* I'm ravenous. I try snacking on grapefruit and salt-free rice cakes, and I give myself pep talks, and I manage to stay on the diet. That self-control makes me feel great.

3) *Sleepless nights.* I'm told to nap in the afternoon. I've never been able to nap during the day. But I try. I lie on the couch and listen to music, and although I don't sleep, I get up feeling better.

4) *Feeling stoned.* I tried pot in college. I inhaled. I got high. I didn't like it. And I don't like this at all. I'm spacey and hyper; my eyes are wide, but my thoughts are empty, yet I'm talking in fast forward. "Prednisone does that," my doctor says when I complain. "Try to deal with it." Do I have a choice?

5) *Stomach pains.* I'm told cortisone can burn a hole in your gut. I am given a strong medication to reduce the acid (Prilosec), and soon I am pain-free. What I am not yet, however, is worry-free. My lung condition could be chronic, I am told, which means even after six months or more on the medication, when I am finally off that medication the disease could return again, and once again, I would have to take major doses of prednisone.

Now I decide that if I am destined to be on this powerful medication for a very long time, I had better arm myself with as much knowledge as possible. I am determined to understand exactly how the drug works and what it can do, to learn about its positive and negative effects. And, as usual, I turn to Julie to teach me.

4

Tell Me in Plain English, What Is This Stuff and Why Do I Need It?

Eugenia and Julie *This chapter is intended as a primer about glucocorticoids, how they work and why they are used.*

Eugenia (E):   What is this medicine? Where does it come from?
Julie (J):   You're taking prednisone, the most commonly prescribed steroid, and it's related to natural steroids called glucocorticoids made by your adrenal glands. But you are going to need to take it in *much* larger amounts than your own adrenals could possibly make in order to get your illness under control.
E: So what is a steroid?
J: Steroids are actually a large group of compounds named for

their common chemical structure (the basis of such compounds is shown in Figure 1a, and one specific compound, that of cortisol, is shown in figure 1b). When you look at the basic structure (Figure 1a), you can see that it has four rings; it's called a 4-ringed structure. Now look at the structure of cortisol (Figure 1b). You can see that it has those four rings, but it also has some additional carbon (C), hydrogen (H), and oxygen (O) atoms attached, which make the structure cortisol. Steroids include compounds called sterols and a large variety of hormones, as well as other substances called glycosides. While these substances are all chemically related to each other by their common four-ringed structure, they differ from each other because of additional carbon atoms or unique chemical changes that lend specific features to each steroid component. Humans and other animals produce many steroids with a wide variety of actions. Such steroids range from cholesterol (from which other steroids are made), to the adrenal gland steroids— glucocorticoids and mineralocorticoids—to sex steroids such as progesterone, estrogen, and androgen, and to vitamins such as vitamin D. In the Appendix of this book, you can look at a few figures that show the way these steroids are synthesized in the human body.

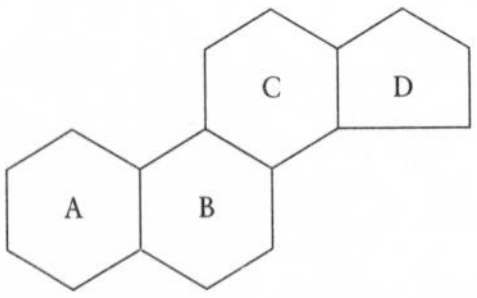

FIGURE 1A

The Four-Ringed
Structure of Steroids

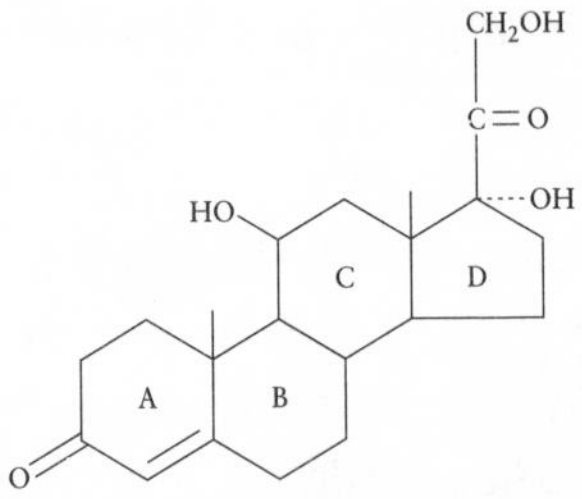

FIGURE 1B

Cortisol

E: How many kinds of steroids are there that a patient could take?

J: A large number, as you can see in the tables found in "Steroids: Types, Potency, Brands." For the purposes of most discussions, doctors say a patient is "on steroids" or "on glucocorticoids." I'll use the term *steroids* or *prednisone* while I talk to you about it.

E: Who invented it?

J: Nobody invented steroids, unless you mean God. Steroids were discovered. And Dr. Philip Hench, who led the group that started using steroids in patients, won the Nobel Prize, because the effects revolutionized the care of many patients with a multitude of problems.

E: Tell me more about this.

J: The modern use of steroids in clinical medicine began just a bit under fifty years ago, in 1949, when a group of doctors at the Mayo Clinic reported the use of cortisone to treat a small group of nine patients with rheumatoid arthritis. The crippling joint stiffness in these nine individuals improved almost miraculously, and a new era in medicine began.

Over the decades that have followed that first report from the Mayo Clinic, pharmaceutical companies have produced a variety of synthesized steroids to be used as medication. Steroids have revolutionized the treatment of many conditions, ranging from rheumatoid arthritis to asthma to kidney diseases to organ transplantation.

E: Why do most doctors prescribe prednisone?

J: The reason that your doctor picked prednisone is that there has been a lot of experience using it for conditions like yours. The side effects that prednisone can cause are well described, and these are fewer than those associated with some other steroid preparations. Furthermore, prednisone is a longer-acting form of steroids than cortisol or cortisone, so that you don't have to take it many times per day. Prednisone is not naturally made in your body, but it is very similar to the steroids that your adrenals make.

E: I'm really worried about the side effects. Are you sure I really need to take it?

J: You do. You have a serious lung disease (eosinophilic pneumonitis) involving a huge amount of inflammation. With eosinophilic pneumonitis, steroids are the mainstay of treatment and improve the outcome. There's a microscopic battle going on in your lungs, and steroids will stop the mayhem. The bottom line is that you have a medical problem that responds to steroids. You'll need a course of high-dose steroids for weeks, months, or maybe years.

E: What questions did my doctor ask himself in order to decide to prescribe prednisone? There are so many medicines, I can't believe there isn't something with fewer side effects.

J: In the near future there may be something else that you could take, but right now steroids are the only option. Of course your doctor asked himself questions. I imagine his thoughts went like this:

How serious is Eugenia's problem? *Very.*

Are steroids the best treatment? *Yes, the outcome is usually better with steroids, and for Eugenia steroids are the only treatment.*

What type of steroids should be used? *She needs steroids that will enter her bloodstream and go to her lungs. This means I'll prescribe them either by mouth or intravenously (IV). But since IV medication necessitates a needle and other hardware, I'll reserve that for emergencies and prescribe pills. I know that steroid aerosols can get into the lungs, but they won't work well here.*

What dose does she need? *From experience with eosinophilic pneumonitis, I'd say she'll need high-dose steroids to start with.*

How long will she need the steroids? *Until her disease is put into remission or cured and the inflammation decreases. After*

that point her dose can be tapered down and possibly stopped.
Will the steroids interact with other medicines that she may need? *Steroids do interact with some other medications, so I'll need to ask her what other drugs she takes. I'll also need to think about this whenever I prescribe any other medication for her.*

Are there individual factors that could influence her response to steroids or cause major side effects? *Yes. If she has conditions such as diabetes mellitus, osteoporosis, certain gastrointestinal problems [peptic ulcer, gastritis, esophageal reflux], chronic infections that would be worsened by steroids [tuberculosis, for example], high blood pressure or heart disease, or psychological difficulties, she may have to be watched especially closely.*

What can be done to try to prevent side effects? *She needs to become educated about the effects of steroids, their probable side effects, especially those that can be anticipated.* (These are discussed in other chapters.)

E: So you say I have to take steroids. Easy for you to say. But how do I decide that I agree?

J: Simple. If you don't, for your problem, Eugenia, your lungs will likely get worse, and you could even die. It is that serious. I know that you'd like to be part of the decision, and you should be. But your condition is life-threatening. There really is *no* choice.

E: What if it weren't so serious? What about patients who don't have a life-threatening disease? How do they make their choices?

J: Supposing their doctor says, "A lot of evidence suggests that steroids are very likely to slow the progression of your disease, but there are no guarantees. If nothing is done, your condition almost surely will get worse." In this case steroids will probably work, slowing or stopping their disease, *but not for sure.* In this case, their decision should be an informed one in which they and their family play a major role.

E: How would that work?

J: Here is an example. Supposing a patient has a kind of kidney disease called membranoproliferative glomerulonephritis. This is one of several forms of chronic and progressive inflammation of the kidney filters (glomeruli) that appear to be steroid-responsive. In that case most doctors would suggest that the decision to use steroids should be based on the likelihood of personal response weighed against the likely problems from taking from the steroids ("the risks") compared to the improvement if the disease gets treated ("the benefits"). In some forms of glomerulonephritis, getting worse means scarred kidneys and kidney failure that can necessitate dialysis or transplant. In this situation, most patients would decide to use steroids.

Sometimes when the disease is not life-threatening, even though the patient knows that steroids will help his or her condition, the decision is *not* to take the steroids. For example, I know of a patient with a chronic skin rash that is unsightly and uncomfortable. She hates the rash. She's been told that nothing else will work as well as steroids; but just as you do, she worries about the side effects. She decided not to take steroids right now. Later, if she decides to take them, she will likely do so on a time-limited basis, during which she and her doctor will monitor her response.

E: How do doctors monitor the patient's response?

J: They observe how the disease responds and weigh that against the side effects. With steroids, most side effects are obvious. For example, the patient would report weight gain, change in mood, visual problems, stomach pain, et cetera. If the side effects become unacceptable, then the medicine can be tapered and eventually stopped, unless the disease is so serious that patient and doctor decide living with the side effects is a lot better than any alternative.

E: Do some people have a greater risk of getting side effects than others?

J: Yes. For instance, some patients have diabetes, and the control of diabetes is usually harder on steroids. Other medications would be discussed, but steroids might still be the best choice.

E: What does that do to that person's diabetes?

J: Their diabetes might require more insulin for the blood sugar to stay controlled. This can be tricky to treat, but it is often done.

E: How does a doctor decide what kind of steroids to prescribe?

J: You should discuss this with your doctor. A good rule of thumb is that the least potent form, with the most direct effect to solve your particular health problem, will be key.

E: Once I begin my course of steroids, how does the medicine get to the right place in my body?

J: The medical phrase *route of administration* refers exactly to that. Medications can be given right into the bloodstream, intravenously, in which case the medicine doesn't need to be absorbed from your intestinal tract, through your skin, or from your lungs. Long courses of steroids are not usually given this way. Usually steroids are given in pill form for serious illnesses like yours. Though steroids can be put into your rectum, put on your skin, and/or inhaled, pills will be more effective. The steroids will be absorbed and then will circulate throughout your body to reach the injured cells that need the most help—in your case, in your lungs.

E: But you said that steroids can be inhaled. Why can't I just use an inhaler?

J: Because the cause of your lung inflammation isn't just locally in your lungs. You have a problem throughout your body that is manifesting itself in your lungs. You need to be treated with steroids that can get both to your lungs and to the cells causing the inflammation.

E: So when will I know if the medicine is working?

J: Whether or not it is effective will be determined by the amount of the medicine you take (dose), how well you absorb it (if you take it by mouth), where it goes in your body (distribution), and how fast you get rid of it (elimination). These factors constitute what is called pharmacokinetics.

E: What do you mean by "elimination"?

J: Steroids don't just stay in your body. They are broken down, or "metabolized," in your liver and kidneys. They are excreted in your urine. One dose of the medicine generally lasts for a number of hours. But the effects can last for much longer.

E: How long does prednisone stay in my body?

J: Each dose will last about half a day. Whether what you take actually gets absorbed from your intestines into your body depends on several factors.

E: Such as?

J: Most steroids don't dissolve very well in water. The amount of food and other material in your stomach may affect absorption. However, if there is edema of your bowel (swelling from extra body water) or diarrhea or constipation, the efficiency of absorption will be affected.

How long the medicine stays around also depends on how your body handles it. Once you take a dose of prednisone, which is actually an inactive form of steroid, it has to be activated in your body. Prednisone (inactive) is converted to prednisolone (active), but some is converted back again into prednisone. So you can see that if a lot of the activated medication is converted back to the inactive drug, it would have less of an effect in your body. Some people convert steroids to the more active forms more efficiently than others. For example, people with some kinds of liver disease are not as efficient at converting the inactive drug to the active compound. For them, taking a form of steroids that is already activated is best.

E: Don't my adrenal glands produce steroids that are a lot like prednisone?

J: Yes, but the pills you are taking will provide much higher levels of steroids in your body and will interrupt the usual way your adrenal glands function.

E: Are you saying that while I am on prednisone my own adrenals shut down?

J: Yes. Steroids that you take as medicine interrupt the way your body's adrenal glands make natural steroids under normal circumstances, and this means that it takes time for the adrenals to function well again.

E: Is that why steroids have to be tapered? Why can't I just stop them when my problem is under control?

J: Your adrenal glands normally make steroids in response to signals from the pituitary, the so-called master gland at the base of your brain. Taking big doses of steroids will interrupt these signals, so that your adrenals will be unable to respond to your body's normal need for steroids. This interruption, often called suppression, can last for weeks and months, and can be responsible for some of the symptoms of withdrawal from steroids. It is one reason why the doses of long-term steroids need to be tapered down gradually rather than stopped "cold turkey." [This is discussed in chapter 11.]

E: I've been told that I'm supposed to take my prednisone in the morning. Why?

J: Your adrenals normally produce steroids in higher amounts in the early hours of the morning. It's thought that if you take your medicine in the morning, you'll be giving steroids in a normal daily pattern. The time of day at which you take glucocorticoids may influence your body's handling of the medication. Higher concentrations are achieved in the body after early-morning doses than evening doses. This may be due to the combined effect of slow elimination of morning doses and decreased absorption of doses in the evening.

E: What happens if one morning I miss a dose? Can I take it later in the day? Or should I take twice the number of pills the next morning?

J: It would be fine to take your pills later the same day. It probably would be better to do that than to take a double dose the next day.

E: In the past, when I've had to take antibiotics, I've been told to avoid alcohol. Do I need to do that now? Are there things that I shouldn't eat or drink when I'm on steroids?

J: You don't need to avoid alcohol, but since prednisone can irritate your stomach, the fact that alcohol also can irritate your stomach should be remembered. Technically, you don't have to avoid any particular foods. (However, because steroids are associated with weight gain and fluid retention, we will provide helpful diet guidelines that combat these side effects.)

E: Is there anything about my particular illness that will affect how steroids will work for me?

J: Not for you, but for some patients with other diseases, the illness itself can affect the way steroids are handled in the body. For example, severe liver disease and hypothyroidism are two conditions that impair corticosteroid elimination. In contrast, hyperthyroidism and certain renal disorders are sometimes associated with accelerated corticosteroid elimination. Some other conditions, such as asthma, do not seem to influence the way the body handles steroids.

E: What if I get a cold and need other medications on top of the steroids?

J: You'll need to take them. But you need to remember that some other medicines can interact with steroids. Some medicines affect the so-called microsomal enzyme system and change how steroids are eliminated from the body. Thus concomitant administration of certain drugs, such as phenobarbital, phenytoin, carbamazepine, ephedrine, and rifampin, may hasten steroid elimination. This means that the effective level of the steroid in your body will be relatively lower when you are on such medications. On the other hand, the use of certain antibiotics in the class called macrolides, such as erythromycin and troleandomycin, may be associated with decreased elimination of methylprednisolone (but not prednisolone).

Some medications can bind steroid doses in your intestine

so that the steroids are not well absorbed. For example, antacids such as Tums can decrease steroid availability, probably by physical absorption (binding) of the steroid to the antacid. Thus antacid doses should be taken separately from the steroid doses.

Oral contraceptives may increase steroid effect because the steroids leave the body more slowly and the steroids are bound to proteins that circulate in the blood. In other words, the medicine stays around longer in people taking oral contraceptives.

It is important to review all the medications you take with your doctor to be sure that they don't interact with each other in a manner that will change the effectiveness of your treatment. When new medications are added, it is wise to review potential interactions of the new medications with the steroids (and vice versa).

E: Is there anything that I can do to control how well the steroids will work?

J: There are individual factors that can influence the effectiveness of the steroids. First, there are the biological factors I've just described. Then, how accurately and consistently you take the medication will, of course, affect how well it works. It is crucial to discuss your willingness and commitment to taking steroids with your doctor. This is not a casual drug, and taking it inconsistently can be very dangerous, even fatal.

E: Are you saying I'll die if I miss a dose?

J: No, of course not. But consistent compliance is crucial.

E: It's good to have you as my private hot line for questions. What would I do if I didn't have an on-line sister who is a doctor?

J: You would keep a notebook for questions as you think of them. If you had an urgent question that couldn't wait, you'd call your doctor. But if the question was not pressing, you could carry the list to your next doctor's appointment.

E: Besides my disease, how many other kinds of illnesses are treated with steroids?

J: The list of conditions for which steroids are prescribed is long and always growing. The box at the end of this chapter lists many such medical problems.

E: What about illnesses in which your own body produces excess steroids. What's that?

J: There are conditions where the body does make much too much glucocorticoid. When this occurs, the physical findings are a lot like those seen when someone is placed on megadoses of steroids. The treatment for overproduction of steroids depends on the cause. The name for this situation is Cushing's syndrome, and people with this problem develop symptoms similar to though often more pronounced than those seen from large doses of steroids prescribed as medicine.

E: What if I suffer a trauma like a car accident or have to have an operation while I'm on long-term steroids? Will the medicine add to my woes?

J: I'm glad you brought this up, because it is really important to remember that big stresses like those you just mentioned should trigger your adrenal glands to make more steroids. But when you are taking large doses of glucocorticoids or have been on these medications for a long time, your adrenal glands can't respond well to signals of stress. So you will need "stress dose" coverage—in other words, a temporary increase in your dose. The booster doses can be given by vein or by mouth, depending on the rest of your medical situation. Then, as soon as practical and safe, the dose is tapered right back down to what you were taking. Most often, the stress doses are given only for one to three days.

You should consider getting a Medic-Alert bracelet or necklace so that if you were injured or suddenly ill, the emergency team would find out about your being on steroids right away. You should also carry a card in your wallet with a list of your medications and a brief note about your illness.

E: I still don't like these steroids! Are any new steroid preparations being developed that will decrease the toxicity that patients have to endure?

J: That certainly is a goal for the future. There are good strategies being studied: For example, it's possible to hook (conjugate) the medication to "linkers" that can be attached to support systems like dextrans that slow how the steroid drug is metabolized. Such preparations are promising because they don't suppress the body's adrenals as much. Another strategy is finding novel ways to get the medication where it is most needed. When possible, local delivery of steroids, as in inhalers or topical preparations, can avoid side effects, though new preparations would need to be developed that are more effective and less toxic than the ones presently available.

E: How can you doctors prescribe something with such mega–side effects?

J: I think that most doctors (and I would hope all) balance the need for every medicine with the risks of using it. All medications have side effects, and I know that sounds trite. I agree with you: steroids do have major side effects. The reason doctors prescribe them, however, is that steroids have miraculously positive effects on a variety of diseases that would otherwise have worse outcomes. The issue is how to address the expected and common side effects and minimize them. I think we all—both doctors and patients—need to keep that in the front of our minds.

Specific Indications for Prednisone

(Adapted from Physicians Desk Reference; McEvoy JK, AHFS 96 American Society of Health-System Pharmacists, AHFS Publishing, 1996.)

Note: Additional indications exist but are not formally FDA-approved. The indications for other forms of glucocorticoids may differ. So, if your condition is not on this list, the indication for steroid use for you or your family member is something you should discuss with your doctor.

Endocrine: adrenal insufficiency, congenital adrenal hyperplasia, severe hypercalcemia, thyroiditis.

Collagen Diseases: systemic lupus erythematosis, systemic polymyositis, acute rheumatic carditis.

Rheumatic Diseases: ankylosing spondylitis, acute and subacute bursitis, acute nonspecific tenosynovitis, acute gouty arthritis, post-traumatic osteoarthritis, epicondylitis.

Skin (Dermatologic) Diseases: pemphigus, bullous dermatitis herpetiformis, severe erythema multiforme, exfoliative dermatitis, mycosis fungoides, psoriasis, severe seborrheic dermatitis (also see "allergic states").

Allergic States: Control of severe or incapacitating allergic conditions intractable to adequate trials of conventional treatment. Seasonal or perennial allergic rhinitis, bronchial asthma, contact dermatitis, atopic dermatitis, serum sickness, drug hypersensitivity reactions.

Eye Diseases: Severe acute and chronic allergic and inflammatory processes involving the eye and its adnexa, for example: Allergic corneal marginal ulcers, herpes zoster of the eye, inflammation of the anterior chamber of the eye, diffuse posterior uveitis and choroiditis, sympathetic ophthalmia, allergic conjunctivitis, keratitis, chorioretinitis, optic neuritis, iritis and iridocyclitis.

Specific Indications for Prednisone, cont.

Lung Diseases: Symptomatic sarcoidosis, Loeffler's syndrome not manageable by other means, berylliosis, disseminated tuberculosis when used concurrently with appropriate antituberculosis chemotherapy, aspiration pneumonitis.

Hematologic Disorders: idiopathic thrombocytopenic purpura (ITP), acquired autoimmune hemolytic anemia, erythroblastopenia, congenital (erythroid) hypoplastic anemia.

Neoplastic Diseases: for the palliative management of leukemias and lymphomas in adults and acute leukemia of childhood.

Edematous States: To induce a diuresis or remission of proteinuria in the nephrotic syndrome (without renal failure) or that due to lupus erythematosis.

Gastrointestinal Diseases: Ulcerative colitis, regional enteritis, liver diseases.

Nervous System: Acute exacerbations of multiple sclerosis, myasthenia gravis.

Renal Diseases: Various nephropathies, nephrotic syndrome, interstitial nephritis.

Transplantation: Solid organ transplants, bone marrow transplants.

AIDS: To act as an adjunct in certain AIDS-related complications.

Miscellaneous: Tuberculous meningitis with blockage to drainage of fluid (when used together with appropriate antituberculosis chemotherapy), bacterial meningitis, trichinosis with neurological or heart involvement, acute spinal cord injury, shock states, chemotherapy-induced vomiting.

5

Depression—
Singing
the Blues

NOTE: *People on prednisone commonly experience mood changes. Some have severe mood swings. Others experience depression or euphoria. Some notice nothing. This is Eugenia's story.*

Eugenia Two weeks into prednisone therapy. I am now a sleepless zombie. My eyes don't focus. I can't concentrate very well. And my emotional roller coaster is making me, and my nearest and dearest, half crazy. My two daughters, Arianna and Natalia, are in their early twenties, and I don't want them to be worried about me. But we're so bonded, they know I'm a wreck without my having to tell them, and now I'm worried that they're worried. Then there is David Seltzer, my filmmaker husband, whom I adore. But he is a man with four adult children from a previous marriage, and his work dominates his life. He is having problems of his own, both professional and parental, and I fear he cannot really "be there" for me. I decide that this battle with prednisone is going to be my own, and as I defend myself for the fight, I feel isolated and glum.

"You think you're depressed?" a former long-term prednisone taker commiserates with me. "I freaked out. I was positively psychotic on the stuff."

I have yet to freak. But it may be in my future. What I am is emotionally fragile. One minute I'm blue, the next I'm hyper and happy. Sometimes I have motor-mouth and I rattle on to anyone who will listen. Other times I am silent as a stone and just as animated. Nonetheless, I'm functional. I practice the flute every day for several hours. I have managed to do some interviews in New York for my CBS TV job and acquit myself adequately. And I have even had one all-day photographic shoot for the cover of an upcoming CD, at which I stared into the lens like a moose caught in headlights while the photographer clicked away, trying to make the most of his glazed subject.

My initial euphoria at finding out what was wrong with me and how to fix it has definitely faded. I find myself worrying about everything. I talk to my husband, who tries to be supportive, and to friends, but mostly I keep my anxieties to myself. Like anyone stricken with a serious illness, I feel a mixture of fear, anger, and isolation. And although I am told my illness is curable, I fantasize about getting worse or having a chronic condition and losing my livelihood. I have been rigorous with my diet, I have exercised, and I am told by my family and friends that I look just the same. There are no visible changes. But inside, I feel like I'm crumbling.

———

Two more weeks pass. Now I'm a month into my prednisone therapy. I have begun to take sixty milligrams of prednisone every other day. This alternating therapy will, supposedly, minimize the side effects of the drug. Although I am glad for the prospect of minimizing damage to my body, I quickly find that taking the drug on alternating days presents an even more pronounced challenge to my brain. The day I'm on the drug, I'm up and enthusiastic. The day I'm off, I'm way off, down in the dumps, listless. I think everyone is annoyed with me, disappointed in me, and that I am a failure at everything.

At my weekly doctor's appointment, at which I have blood and x-rays taken, I am told that the pulmonary infiltrates are fading nicely. I am also asked how I feel, and I answer, "Well, I can breathe, but I can't sleep; I have mood swings, visual weirdness, depression; I think I'm getting a little paranoid. . . ." With a pat on the arm and a smile, my doctor tells me not to worry, it's the medication, and, after all, the medication is doing its job.

My doctor is not unsympathetic. He is interested in curing my disease. I wonder whether I should be trying harder to communicate my concerns and fears to him, but I don't want to sound like a wimp or impose on his time. And after all, I tell myself, a lung specialist is not a shrink. But when friends suggest that I see a therapist, I resist. I figure that if the mood swing thing is caused by the cortisone, I'll just tough it out until I'm off the stuff.

Two more weeks pass. I am still on sixty milligrams of prednisone every other day. My x-rays show that the disease is retreating. I am feeling strong enough to take my first out-of-town trip—to Houston to do an interview for CBS, then on to Bowling Green, Ohio, where I will perform for the first time in over a month. I decide to stop in Oberlin, Ohio, en route to Bowling Green to see my younger daughter, Natalia, who is a student at Oberlin College. This trip will be business and pleasure, and I look forward to it. But as I prepare to leave, I begin to experience yet another side effect of prednisone: panic. During the previous month I may have worried and fretted, but *this* is very different. What if I'm in Houston and I can't find my prednisone? What if I can't find fat-free, salt-free foods? What if I'm onstage in Ohio and I can't breathe? An electric shock of fear zips through me at each imagined problem. And as I actually wheel my suitcase toward the waiting taxi, I am overwhelmed with panic: Do I have my pills? Did I pack my gown? Where's my flute? My plane ticket? My wallet?! Each internal question produces a jab of terror, as if someone had come up behind me and screamed into my ear.

On the plane to Houston, the passenger beside me begins to sneeze and cough. My immune system is compromised. I could get sick, as if I'm not sick enough already! I arrive in Houston with a level of anxiety I have never before experienced. The smallest glitch leaves me shaking. I find myself in a hotel room in a state of panic. Of course I realize it must be caused by the prednisone. But each tiny episode of panic, although understood as chemically induced, nonetheless takes a toll. It is not only distressing to be zapped with a sudden rush of fear, but it also requires considerable effort to calm myself down afterward. I pace around my room and talk to myself. I unpack, wash up, and descend to the hotel restaurant to join my CBS producer and crew for dinner.

In the restaurant, I manage to find the right foods to eat. Not only have I had six weeks on prednisone practicing making special requests in New York restaurants, but it seems that these days eateries across the country are becoming accustomed to all kinds of dietary demands. Of course the colleagues with whom I'm dining want to know what's up, why the weird requests. They are not satisfied with, "I'm on some strong medication." They want to know the whole story, and I tell it, reluctantly, assuring them that my disease is rare and it is neither bacterial nor viral and therefore they cannot catch it. But midstory I panic. Will the word get out that I've got this disease? Will I lose my television job? And if it becomes known in the world of music, who will hire a flutist with a lung disease? My colleagues are very compassionate, but nonetheless, I can't sleep.

I get out of bed early to go over the extensive information I have for my interview with the conductor of the Houston Symphony, Christoph Eschenbach—press releases, magazine articles, reviews. But my mind is muddled. I can't seem to concentrate. And I can't remember the kinds of details that I normally retain like a sponge. *Not to worry,* I tell myself. I've known Christoph for a long time, and even if I can't read the materials, I should easily be able to interview him.

I arrive at Christoph's book-and-art-filled apartment that overlooks the city, excited to see him again, but I'm anxious. I am proud of my ability to interview my subjects without notes and with a musician's sensibility—listening well, letting my subject's answer lead me to my next question. But will I be able to concentrate on what I'm hearing? As Christoph and I sit down in front of the cameras, I panic. I can't even think what to ask first. The cameras roll. Somehow I begin, and it is Christoph's gentle spirit and brilliant mind that inspire me, help me focus.

Everyone is pleased. I'm in a great mood. I have a quick salt-free lunch, and I'm off to the airport to fly to Ohio, where I will stop overnight in Oberlin to visit Natalia. I know how concerned she is about me, and I want to appear healthy and relaxed. But as I get into her car at the Cleveland airport, I see cat hairs on the seats and I panic—my disease, eosinophilic pneumonitis, is triggered by an allergic response, and although the "trigger" is very difficult to pinpoint, my doctor feels that cats are one possible source of the disease. So there I am, with my beloved child, surrounded by some possibly harmful hairs and trying not to let her see my fear. By early evening I can feel my face fall, my mood plummet.

Sensitive to her mother's every move, Natalia asks, "What's wrong?"

And I say, "I'm just tired. It's been a long day. And my medication is making me a little loopy."

I can feel her worry. And because I wanted to assure rather than alarm her, I go to my motel room feeling guilty and morose.

After some sleep, I wake up the next morning and I manage to be bubbly at breakfast. I kiss Natalia good-bye, telling her not to worry—I'm absolutely fine. And I'm off to play my concert in Bowling Green, warmed with her golden glow. But passing a car on a two-lane road with plenty of room to spare makes my alarms ring. I begin to sweat. Then, getting onto the interstate is a fright fest. And I arrive at my destination, exhausted and feeling blue.

At Bowling Green State University I'm giving a concert with the Shanghai Quartet. I'm delighted to see my colleagues—four terrific young men. My mood is up! We rehearse, and all goes well. But then, dressed and prepared for the concert, I'm jumpy and anxious. My normal performance style is controlled and relatively relaxed. Of course there are times when I'm nervous onstage, but until now I have never experienced this—utter panic! I see a note. It's an F. Or is it an F sharp? Instant terror attacks me, as if someone had jumped me in a dark alley. My heart races; I feel my head spin. And I experience these little panic attacks throughout the performance. After the concert, I am astonished when everyone says I played well. We celebrate with a late meal, and even though I congratulate myself on successfully getting through my trip, I go to bed feeling blue. I remember my friend who said she was positively psychotic on "the stuff." I begin to think I'm at the edge of that cliff, too, clinging to sanity by my fingertips.

I return to New York exhausted. I try to rest. But I have so much work to do, CBS work, and concerts the following week and the week after that. In fact, I have concerts booked through the following two years. The thought terrifies me. How will I live with the level of anxiety I experienced onstage in Ohio? How will I weather the panic and the outrageous mood swings?

At the doctor's office a few days later, my blood tests come back with a marked increase in eosinophils. This is bad, I am told. This is serious. This means my disease is not responding to taking the medication every other day. I will now have to take fifty milligrams of prednisone one day, ten the next, et cetera.

"Will the side effects get worse?" I ask.

"We'll just have to see," says the doctor, looking somber.

I experience a flash of rage. It's not the doctor's fault. I know that. But still, I'm in a fury, the force of which I know is irrational, but there it is anyhow. Now I begin to be snappish at home. I'm annoyed at my husband for the slightest thing. Small events begin to set me off, for example, the telephone: Wrong-number calls can make me slam the receiver down in a rage, instead of my usual polite, "I'm sorry, but I think you've dialed incorrectly." Being put on hold, usually a mild annoyance to us all, makes me go ballistic. "You've left me dangling for ten minutes!" I fume at someone's secretary, when it probably has been three. "Put me through, now!"

These minitantrums are uncontrollable. They come out of nowhere, like little tornadoes, swirl through me, and disappear, leaving me dazed by my own response. I try to take charge of these outbursts. I tell myself, "Back off; you're on prednisone." Sometimes the reminder works, and sometimes it doesn't. I'm not good at forgiving myself. I fear I am becoming someone else. Someone I don't know. And that frightens and depresses me.

Julie By most standards, Eugenia *didn't* have florid psychiatric side effects from her prednisone treatment. But she wasn't acting much like the sister I've known forever. She was touchy, obsessed with details. For instance, it so happened that she was thinking of changing to a different pulmonologist (lung expert). She was practically trembling with worry about this un-derstandable switch. Would the first doctor be angry at her? What would he do about this great insult? Would the new doc-tor be as competent as everyone said? Would he be sufficiently empathic? What if she didn't like him? Would doctor number one take her back? Would the new doctor mess up and not taper her medication fast enough? Would he taper it inappropriately fast? Again, was he competent? Would he curtail her travel ac-tivities? What did I know about him? Could I find out some-thing more? Or couldn't I? I explained that patients switch doctors rather frequently and that doctors can certainly under-stand this. It is no biggie. My thoughts were, *Eugenia has every right to be worried and scared. I'll try to address all of this as well as I can.* However, when your laid-back little sister has sud-denly metamorphosed into a worry whirlwind, it is hard to "get it." One afternoon she called me at work three (3!) times within about twenty minutes to be sure I was going to send her x-rays back to New York to a consultant to whom she was con-sidering switching her care (these had been sent to Boston for review by an infectious diseases expert at my hospital). Euge-nia was sure that now the films were lost, that maybe she'd never get the care she needed, the care that would save her life: "The films aren't here. Why haven't they arrived? You can't be sure that FedEx didn't lose my films, and now the new doctor won't believe I had those infiltrates." She went on and on.

I pretty quickly lost my cool, doctorly manner. *What has got-ten into her?* I wondered. I knew, *Yes, Eugenia is on high-dose steroids. That is probably it.* But I lost my temper anyway. Ex-asperated, I snapped at her. I said something on the order of, "Come on, Genie, I didn't eat the films. Yours are not the first x-rays FedEx ever got. I can check. Get a grip!"

Even now, we each recall The Episode of the x-rays differently. We still discuss all this gingerly. I, the big sister, have always been prone to having a temper at home, despite the cool bedside manner. Genie, the younger sister, has always been more mellow. So whose memory is "right"?

What Eugenia was experiencing with her mood swings is quite typical: Rapid mood swings, change in personality, even if mild, and change in perception of what is happening are all usual when on high-dose steroids. Sleep disturbance is frequently reported, and doctors tell their patients to "live with it" or "drink warm milk at bedtime." Or they may prescribe bedtime sedation. The whys and wherefores for all of these changes are not well understood. "We see this," is what most texts state. As doctors, we don't prepare patients and families adequately. And we don't provide strategies for our patients as a result. Perhaps it is because we don't have the time to listen or because the myriad complaints seem insoluble, unapproachable, and minor compared to the serious medical problems we are trying to treat.

Psychiatric Side Effects of Steroids

What Eugenia was describing is very common. Her psychiatric side effects were quite mild, which is usually the case. But she did not experience her anxiety as mild. She did not anticipate the anxiety, and it upset her. If the doctor only bothers to ask, he or she will learn that most patients on high-dose steroids will report some feelings of being anxious, having mood swings, or noting lack of concentration. Like Eugenia, the patient will say that he or she feels "different," "anxious," "not him/herself," or "easily upset." If family members are really questioned, they will also usually report that the patient is "touchy," "moody," "different." Indeed, over the past four decades the medical literature has described a broad range of psychiatric side effects associated with steroids. In practice, however, doctors minimize such reports, because the beneficial reasons for using steroids generally place the psychiatric side effects in the category of pesky problems, from the doctor's point of view. The reasons to give the steroids usually by far outweigh the effect these medications will have on mood, perception, or even mental stability. So, as practitioners, we concentrate on the illness and mention in passing, at best, that this kind of medicine "may affect your mood." On reflection, I think we do our patients and their families a big disservice by sweeping this type of side effect under the rug. It is very reassuring for people to know that they should *expect* to feel different. Then they won't feel "crazy" and won't feel like stopping the medication cold turkey, which is very dangerous.

In children, side effects range from hyperactivity and irritability with inability to concentrate to anxiety, depression, and withdrawn behavior. This can lead to real difficulty in the school setting, as a child on high-dose steroids may become disruptive in class or may have trouble concentrating on schoolwork. With advance warning, the parents of a child on high-dose steroids can talk to teachers and counselors up front, which can help the child (and the class).

So, my sister's experience with how steroids made her feel has made me a more considerate steroid prescriber.

It is disappointing that few studies have been large enough to begin to document how pervasive a problem this may be. Steroids are now very widely used for a host of indications, but the *actual incidence* of psychiatric side effects is truly unknown. The medical literature describes the psychiatric effects of glucocorticoid therapy as varied and fairly common. It is said that the most common personality changes are reported as "mood changes," mild euphoria to a state of pressured activity known as hypomania. Yet depression, psychosis, and even transitory dementia have been reported. As a clinician who talks to many patients, I think that the effects of steroids on mood, concentration, and perception are vastly underestimated in both adult and pediatric patients.

Some studies suggest that psychiatric side effects while on steroids are proportional to dosage: the more you take, the more likely it will be that you'll have marked side effects. Usually the symptoms lessen with reduction of the dose, generally done as a slow, planned reduction (called tapering), but mood swings and depression are common as high-dose steroids are tapered.

In the worst case scenario, patients become severely affected and develop steroid psychosis or dementia. In such cases, antipsychotic or antianxiety medications may be needed. It is important to note, however, that people often use the phrase *steroid psychosis* loosely, describing patients who are very upset on steroids. In this sense, *steroid psychosis* can be a "bad" label and a true misnomer; in truth, patients rarely become frankly psychotic. Adults may have rapidly alternating mood swings, which will be hard for family and friends to understand.

In the early years of prescribing steroids, two doctors named Dr. H. Rome and Dr. F. Braceland studied a group of patients and their responses to ACTH (the pituitary hormone that makes the adrenal gland release natural steroids), prednisone, hydrocortisone, and related steroid substances. While much has been learned in the forty-four years since their study was published, it is important because it documented the range of effects that can occur: Mild effects in their study occurred in 60 percent of patients. These were reported as euphoria, impaired sleeping and restlessness, and perhaps less good judgment than normal. More severe reactions, including marked obsessional thought, rumination, anxiety, and hypomania, occurred in 25 to 30 percent of the patients. About 10 percent of the patients had true psychosis.

Why Do Steroids Cause Mood Changes?

The reasons for mood swings and other neuropsychological effects of steroids are complex. Some are pragmatically understood, as roller-coaster emotions are natural and to be expected when facing a serious disease. Others may involve neurotransmitters. Here is a straightforward listing:

- *Relief: a factor not directly related to steroids.* The main factor is that someone who needs high-dose steroids is likely to have a serious medical problem. Eugenia was faced with a potentially life-threatening lung condition, which was making her feel like she was gasping for breath on the bottom of a swimming pool. The eosinophilic pneumonitis might, in the most dire circumstance, kill her, or it could stop her career dead in its tracks. She was frightened, depressed, and feeling helpless. Then the steroids made her miraculously better. After a reprieve, one naturally feels relief, euphoria. The same euphoria occurs with responses to other medications, with physical therapy, or even with placebos.

  Very young children also have a lot of mood changes, however, at an age when the gravity of their situation does not impress them. Yes, they feel better, and yet the "relief" factor is probably minor.
- *Effect on brain receptors.* Glucocorticoids (steroids) bind to specific receptors in the brain and may have direct effects.
- *Effect on neurotransmitters.* Glucocorticoids increase release of norepinephrine, serotonin, and other neurotransmitters.
- *Effect in changing hormonal balance between the adrenal-pituitary axis.*

It is fair to say that as steroids have potent effects on cell function, it makes sense that there would be generalized central nervous system effects. Such effects probably should be studied more completely. If you or a family member needs steroids, you need some guidelines, a kind of mapping out of what may happen to your mood or your loved one's mood.

In that light, here's what you should know about the psychological effects of steroids, how you might feel, and what you can do:

- *High-dose steroids.* Be aware that most people will have *some* mood changes while they are on high-dose steroids. These effects are dose-dependent and will lessen later as the medication dose is tapered. For reasons not well understood, some people seem to get these effects almost immediately, while others don't get them at all. Be aware that *most* people really have mild changes. So, you may feel euphoric at first, especially when your medical problem improves, perhaps getting dramatically better. Later you may notice that you feel optimistic one minute and weepy the next. Or irritable or affable. Be lenient with yourself (suggestions about what to do are found below).

- *Steroid taper.* Most people will have periods of feeling very blue while their steroids are being reduced. They may also feel exhausted and intermittently depressed. It is crucial to remind yourself that this is temporary and that the good news is that you are getting better, and thus your medication can be decreased and possibly discontinued altogether.

- *Resumption or increase in dose of steroids after a taper.* If you have to go back on steroids, it brings up all kinds of understandable worries, about the illness itself as well as the side effects. But even if you had serious psychiatric side effects on high-dose steroids before, they will not necessarily recur this time around. Make sure you discuss the situation with your doctor and set up arrangements *in advance* for surveillance and management of the side effects.

Here are some simple suggestions for what to do:

- *Ask that your doctor talk about the psychiatric aspects of high-dose steroids with you.* Be sure that you have worked out a mental checklist, so that if you have unbearable mood swings or anxiety, you can get the help you need. This may simply mean a series of relaxation steps. It may mean using antianxiety medication for a period of time. Such a checklist should provide guidelines about when to consider psychiatric side effects an emergency (be reassured that psychiatric emergencies are very rare indeed).

- *Ask for understanding from your family.* The medicine is indeed a "wonder" drug, but you may have mood swings, be sensitive, and/or irritable. They need to know up front that this is not anything they or you have "done."

- *Avoid stressful situations, if you can.* Many of us, like Eugenia, have demanding work, work that brings us into contact with others in stressful situations. You can't stop work. But you can anticipate. Perhaps you will want to get stress reduction tapes. Perhaps you will want to get counseling for the period of time you are on high-dose medication and tapering it down.

How Widespread Is the Mood Problem?

How prevalent are personality changes when patients take steroids? Frank psychosis from high-dose steroids is blessedly rare. When it occurs, however, it is related neither to dose nor duration of therapy; but symptoms are flamboyant and disturbing. Over the years I have had patients screaming about bugs on the walls or a mild-mannered man claiming to be a gangster who could have someone "rubbed out" for me. A patient who doesn't become frankly psychotic nonetheless can seem like a totally different person, extroverted instead of introverted, for example. Less marked personality changes are common, yet the actual incidence of clear and significant mood change is unreported. My best guess is that *most* patients likely have some perceptible changes in how they feel while on steroids. They may not notice much, or they may feel very "different." They may or may not realize what is going on and usually do not think right away that it is due to the medication.

So, as a physician, I would say:

- Mood swings really *are* expectable. When these occur, remember that they are related to your therapy. You have not turned into someone else. And it will be temporary.
- You can get help in dealing with these viscissitudes:
  1) Use stress reduction techniques.
  2) Use affirmations to calm yourself down.
  3) Be sure your relatives and friends understand and are educated about this.
  4) If these changes are disabling, yet you need to stay on steroids, get the help of a psychopharmacologist, in order to control the symptoms with medication, if necessary.

6

Diet Guidelines: Beating the Bloat and the Munchies

This chapter contains practical and personal advice about eating while on high-dose steroids. It is important to work out your own method for keeping your appetite in check and finding foods you like. A nutritionist can be invaluable. We present this chapter as something that worked for Eugenia. We specifically do not claim that this diet is scientifically proven.

Julie

Why Should You Be on a Special Diet?

Why not just keep on eating as you always have? If you do that, unless your diet is *already* like the one described in this chapter, you are likely to gain some weight, especially if you don't anticipate the possibility of the bloat and the munchies.

Steroid treatment may cause weight gain and redistribution of body fat *even if you watch your diet*. Some people just *do* get more side effects than others. But there is a lot that you can do. Steroids do stimulate the appetite, leading to food-eating rampages of monumental proportions for some people.

You may be thin, fat, or average in weight when you start steroids. If you are already overweight, going on high-dose steroids can worsen the situation.

What Is This Diet?

Eugenia's diet was low in salt, fat, and simple carbohydrates. Such a diet is low in calories but not in essential vitamins and minerals. Eugenia limited other foods, for instance, foods containing yeast. These changes were additions of her own devising that I, as a doctor, can't either refute or support with any authority, but they worked for her.

You should talk with your doctor about the diet plan you devise. You should be sure to tell your doctor and health-care team about changes you make in your eating.

You should also assess your present weight and nutritional status if you change your eating habits. Make realistic goals for yourself. Be sure that any diet will include sufficient vitamins and minerals. There is no harm in taking a multivitamin.

Remember, the weight gain and redistribution seen during steroid therapy *is* likely to be influenced by what you eat. You will need to work out a diet that works for you.

What Is Known about Steroids and Salt, Fats, and Carbohydrates in Your Diet?

Salt   A tendency to fluid retention is a probable side effect of steroids, and sticking to a no-added-salt diet can really help cut down on this problem. High blood pressure is another known side effect from steroids, and a no-added-salt diet may prevent or help to control this problem. The no-added-salt diet is, in any event, completely harmless and well worth the effort it takes to get used to less salt in the diet. In fact, the average American takes in far more salt than necessary.

Fats   Fat has nine calories per gram, compared to four for protein and carbohydrates. So gram for gram and ounce for ounce, fats have more calories. Just on this basis, if you want to lose weight a low-fat diet makes intuitive sense. Furthermore, steroids may lead to increases in levels of blood fat, called hyperlipidemia. The way in which this occurs is complicated, and a low-fat diet may not correct the problem completely. Nonetheless, a diet low in fats, especially low in cholesterol, may help prevent or minimize this problem.

Carbohydrates   Carbohydrates (or sugars and starches) are a major part of our diets. These are available as "simple" or sugary foods or as "complex" carbohydrates that must be broken down by the body before they can be used. The complex carbohydrates are less sweet and are less likely to give you a "sugar high." It has been said that steroid side effects on weight gain and redistribution are aggravated by simple carbohydrates. Finding scientific data to support this contention is just about impossible. I scoured the medical literature to find out where and how this observation was found and what the evidence was. I couldn't. I found "soft data," references within references. However, it is certainly *not* harmful to avoid simple carbohydrates. And it may help prevent the chubby cheeks and upper truncal weight gain that are often associated with steroid use. So while I can't recommend this dietary change on strong scientific grounds, I do recommend it as a practitioner who has observed its positive results.

Going Overboard

Some patients are so terrified of weight gain while taking glucocorticoids that they starve themselves, which can even lead to a kind of pseudo-anorexic state. This is equally or more dangerous than overeating! Such patients are at risk for protein-calorie malnutrition and aggravation of the low total body potassium that glucocorticoids can cause. If you find that you are overdoing weight control or if your doctor thinks so, take it seriously. Be sure that you get counseling from a nutritionist and devise a diet that is isocaloric and healthful.

Finding solid data to support the idea that a diet low in fats, low in processed carbohydrates, and low in salt will prevent some of the side effects from steroids is hard to do. We scoured the medical literature to try to find such information yet came up with almost nothing. We have produced a commonsense, relatively low-calorie diet with adequate protein that is certainly not harmful and may be helpful.

Guidelines for Healthy Eating
No Added Salt

It takes about three months to alter an appetite for salt. Consult the box on page 48 for guidelines in establishing a no-added-salt diet, and consider keeping it as a way of life: It does get easier to comply with the diet as time goes on, and you won't need to re-train your appetite if you ever need to take steroids again.

A Diet Low in Processed Carbohydrates

Finding solid data to support the idea that a diet low in processed, "simple" sugars will cut down on Cushingoid appearance is, frankly, impossible. The references to this exist, to our knowledge, within review articles and so cannot be construed as "scientifically rigorous." However, the idea that avoiding simple, sugary foods will help you in your goal of minimizing the rounded face and fatty trunk figure of someone on high-dose steroids is appealing. At the least, avoiding such foods will provide a more healthful diet, since most of these foods are "junk foods" anyway. The following table gives some examples:

Avoid Foods Containing Simple Carbohydrates such as:	**Eat** Foods Containing Complex Carbohydrates such as:
Hard candies	Rice
Icing	Beans
Chocolate bars	Yams
Twinkies	Couscous

No-Added-Salt Diet Guidelines

Note that while you are on steroids:
Taking less salt in diet will decrease side effects, including high blood pressure.

A no-added-salt diet is not harmful.

Guidelines for such a diet follow

Don't add salt to cooking.

Check food labels, now that labeling is required and content of salt, protein, et cetera, is usually on the labels.

Note: Foods to Avoid
Processed meats such as ham, smoked turkey, hot dogs, salami, pepperoni
Bacon
Smoked salmon and smoked meats
Pickles (and other vegetables in brine)
Salted chips, crackers, pretzels
Many cheeses
Spices that have sodium chloride in them (for example, lemon-salt, celery salt)
Fast foods—unless you specifically ask for no added salt and it is affirmed that the establishment can do it
Dressings: soy sauce, some commercial salad dressings, mustard
Most pizza

Note: Foods to Use
No-salt-added chips, crackers, pretzels
Spices low in salt: pepper, garlic, onion flakes (Note: salt "substitute" has a lot of potassium. This can be a problem for some people. Check about this with your doctor.)
"Pickles" made without salt (see Recipe section)
Lower-salt meats: chicken, turkey, most fish, beef—all if not "preserved."
Fresh fruits and vegetables
Pasta
Rice

Eugenia From day one on prednisone I understand the French expression *faim d'un loup*—hungry as a wolf. That is me. I want to rip into a side of beef, devour an entire cheese cake, down a quart of Ben and Jerry's, crunch a bag of Doritos. I know that prednisone is causing this Rabelasian appetite, but still, I want to eat all day long. I think about food constantly. But I find that frequent snacking (on rice cakes, fruits, vegetables, or unsalted sunflower seeds) takes the edge off my hunger and helps me control my cravings.

But what am I supposed to eat for actual meals? Julie has already given me the following guidelines: no salt, sugar, fats or simple carbohydrates. But does that mean *complete* abstinence from all of the above? I call Julie yet again and ask.

I recall her telling me the following: Most foods contain some salt, but I should not add any while I am on prednisone. I must stay away from sweets not only because they're fattening, but also because diabetes is a possible risk with prednisone and it runs in our family. So, no candy, gum, cakes, chocolate, and all those good things. Fruits are naturally sweet, but I should stay away from the really sweet ones like grapes and bananas and sweetened canned or dried fruits. I can always use sugar substitutes like Equal or Sweet'n Low. I can have olive oil, but I have to keep away from animal fats and red meats. I'll need lots of lean protein, but I should go easy on the pasta and I should probably drink fresh grapefruit juice, because potassium loss is another possible side effect of prednisone. I need calcium-rich foods in order to avoid yet another side effect—bone loss. And I shouldn't forget to eat my vegetables.

I've already taken yeast out of my diet, and Julie tells me I can leave it out if I feel it's helping keep my thrush under control. I decide to stay off yeast. That means no bread, no prepared foods that contain yeast—and there are plenty of those, I discover, as I begin a vigilant label reading of food products I normally buy. And I'm shocked at how much sodium is added to packaged foods. A small portion of Grape Nuts will give me 360 milligrams of sodium. My favorite packaged wheat pilaf contains 650 milligrams per serving. Canned soups, even the supposed low-sodium ones, are out of the ballpark. And I don't even know how much sodium per day the average person consumes. My head spins. How can I figure out what to eat without bothering Julie every three seconds? I consider seeing a nutritionist, but I have consulted several highly recommended ones in the past, for various reasons, and found them too expensive, too ready to put me on repugnant substances that will cleanse my liver or clear my colon, and too eager to sell me vitamins and other supplements. Besides, my doctor has strongly advised that I take *no* over-the-counter medicines or supplements, since it is possible that some compound in one of such remedies may have triggered my disease. I should have no vitamins, minerals, not even painkillers like Tylenol. I am told to take only prednisone, the Prilosec for my stomach, the estrogen that I, recently menopausal, have begun to take for hormone replacement, and calcium supplements to help avoid bone loss.

I decide that there is only one way for me to determine what to eat: I will devise a diet myself. I know the guidelines. Now I will simply take charge of figuring it all out. However, I don't exactly have the time to become the Martha Stewart of the Perfect Prednisone Diet. How can I do this efficiently, without making myself crazy (crazier)?

There must be books about nutrition, I decide, a book that can educate me on food values and content, and eureka! I find one on my very own recipe book shelf in the kitchen: *The Wellness Encyclopedia of Food and Nutrition,* put out by the University of California at Berkeley, with a subtitle: "How to Buy, Store, and Prepare Every Variety of Fresh Food." I have no idea how this book found its way into my kitchen. Maybe it was a gift. Or maybe I actually bought it. But I have never opened this beautifully illustrated tome before, and instantly it becomes my food Bible.

I turn to chapter 1, the "Nutrition Directory." I thought I knew what simple carbohydrates are. But I realize how ill-informed I am as I read: "Simple carbohydrates are the sugars. . . . [T]here are dozens of sugars . . . fructose, glucose, maltose, lactose . . . ," and they "turn up in some unlikely places—processed foods such as soups, spaghetti sauces, fruit drinks, frozen dinners, cereals, and yogurts, as well as in breads, condiments, canned goods, and, of course, soft drinks and what we call 'sweets.' Sugar also occurs naturally in fruits, vegetables and dairy products." Now I realize that I'll have to be even more vigilant about processed food intake, and as Julie has already suggested, I'll stick to naturally sweetened foods, and not too much even of that.

I begin to browse further into the encyclopedia's pages. I find that red peppers have three times as much vitamin C as an orange and that vitamin D and lactose (milk sugar) help improve calcium absorption by the body, whereas oxalic acid, found in vegetables like spinach, actually reduces the absorption ability. Parsnips have a lot of potassium. So do chestnuts, and they are the only nut that is low in fat and calories. Jerusalem artichokes have more than three times the iron of an equal serving of broccoli. Cheeses are even higher in sodium content than I imagined. I see that 3 1/2 ounces of blue cheese has 1,395 milligrams of sodium; Roquefort, 1,809 milligrams. I then check the book's recommended dietary allowances chart, and sodium is listed, for the average person, at "no more than 2400mg." A serving of blue cheese or Roquefort has more than half the allotted daily amount for the normal person. I love cheese. But I am no longer normal. So what do I do? I know I need my dairy products, so instead of eating cheeses, I decide to stick to skim milk and plain nonfat yogurt, both relatively low in sodium content. I will also make "yogurt cheese," a simple task.

As I peruse the book in my spare moments, gathering information, I begin to feel a sense of responsibility and ownership.

Prednisone has invaded my body, but I will fight its side effects by taking charge of a diet that may protect me from some of them. There is little I feel in control of right now except this diet. And I am actually enjoying the process of figuring it out.

The regime I ended up devising for myself may not work for anyone else. But for the ten months that I spent first taking and then tapering down from high doses of glucocorticoids, this diet (coupled with exercise) helped me keep my weight down. I was highly motivated, but I also never felt deprived. Once I became accustomed to eating less sweet and less salty foods, I stopped craving them. I never felt unduly tempted to indulge in some of my preprednisone passions such as candies, sweet muffins, salty smoked salmon, pickles. With the guidance of the *Wellness Encyclopedia*, I began to feel exactly that—*well*. There was also additional helpful nutritional advice that I gathered from eclectic sources. Ira Lieberman, the chiropractor who keeps my flute-challenged spine in alignment, told me to eat a yam a day. "Yams," he said, "are a source of natural cortisone." Although there was no reference to the steroid properties of yams in the encyclopedia, I duly noted that I could get 20,063 IUs of vitamin A from one sweet potato, that they are not terribly caloric, and that, according to the *Wellness Encyclopedia*, "these tuberous roots are among the most nutritious foods in the vegetable kingdom." I decided I could not go wrong, and from then on, the yam became a staple of my diet—a plain baked (microwaved) yam, sprinkled with black pepper or sometimes with cinnamon. Even now, postprednisone, a yam sends me to breakfast heaven.

Arthur Wooten, the shiatsu genius whom I see on occasion, told me that there are four foods that act as natural diuretics—garlic, parsley, asparagus, and grapefruit. Since I happen to like all four of those items, I simply ate more of them. And when I was in withdrawal from prednisone, dragged down with crushing fatigue, it was Arthur who said, "Eat licorice. It jazzes the adrenals." I stopped into my local candy shop and found an article from the *New York Post* (dated the week of 6/3/94) taped to the counter extolling the virtues of licorice. "A drug made from the licorice extract . . . shows promise in preventing common cancers," I read. "It prevents skin tumors . . . has potential for fighting viruses and bacteria as well as stimulating the immune system. . . . [T]he Japanese use it to treat HIV. . . ." Even though no claim was made in the article regarding its stimulation of the adrenals, I buy sugar-free low-salt shiny black stuff and chomp. I'm instantly jazzed. Julie later informed me that licorice contains a steroid-like substance that causes hypertension if eaten in large amounts, but in small amounts was safe.

What part suggestion played I cannot say, but I do know that many of the nutritional tips offered to me from various sources seemed to help enormously.

The diet I crafted was personal and subjective. I followed it faithfully during my high-dose prednisone therapy and during withdrawal from it . . . and after, just because I liked it and it made me feel well. Here is a skeletal summary of the diet, offered in the hopes that it may help others on prednisone with the process of figuring out how to beat the munchies and the bloat (for actual recipes, see chapter 14).

EZ's Prednisone Diet Plan

(NOTE: *Because I put myself on a yeast-free diet, I did not have breads, crackers, et cetera, or fermented foods, such as vinegar, wine, et cetera, which add to yeast build up. This was a self-imposed limitation. But most breads and crackers have sugars and salt in them, and most patients will want to limit consumption for those reasons.*)

Snacks

I snacked at frequent intervals in order to mute the munchies.
I carried salt-free rice cakes with me.

   Other snacks: Fruits. Cucumbers. Carrots. Cherry tomatoes.
Sugar-free and salt-free candies.

Grazing

Instead of three large meals, I often ate smaller portions spread
out over the day to help quell my constant hunger.

Condiments

I used no salt in cooking but added plenty of other spices. I
chopped up fresh ginger and garlic, mixed it together, kept a
container of it stored in the refrigerator and put it in salads, vegetables, chicken, and fish. I bought salt-free blends of spices and
herbs, available in small containers from spice sections in all
food stores. I carried them with me on trips. I squeezed lemon
(sometimes lime) and sprinkled black pepper on almost everything.

Fats

I cooked only with vegetable oil, mostly olive, and used it sparingly. My favorite salad dressing was olive oil and lemon, with
garlic, ginger, and pepper. Luckily my husband liked it, too. He
found that my salt-free cooking was so tasty that he never added
table salt.

Breakfast Choices

1 large yam sprinkled with pepper or cinnamon
or
plain nonfat yogurt (sometimes Dannon light—flavored with
Nutrasweet) and a few plain unsalted rice cakes
or
grapefruit and a boiled egg and rice cakes
or
hot rolled oats or any other hot or cold cereal that does not contain high sodium or sugar content, with some berries on top
or
fresh berries or other fruits that are not excessively sweet. I ate
a lot of kiwis, cantaloupe, grapefruit. I varied the fruits.

Lunch Choices

Because I did not eat bread, I never had sandwiches but satisfied myself with either:
yogurt or yogurt cheese, with fruits or vegetables (fresh or
frozen, microwaved briefly) and rice cakes
or
plain grilled boneless, skinless chicken breast (or plain grilled
fish) with simple cooked or uncooked vegetables
or
Egg white vegetable omelette
or
a small no-salt-added can of sardines, tuna, or salmon (all have
high calcium content) on top of a mixed salad (oil and lemon
dressing)

Dinner

chicken or fish, simply grilled or broiled with vegetables; rice without salt or a plain baked potato (no butter, but lots of pepper and sometimes lemon)

or

pasta tossed with olive oil and garlic or with vegetables. I found no-salt-added tomato pureed products and sometimes cooked with them. Mixed berries or other fruit for dessert.

Coffees, Teas, and Soda

I was told to limit coffee intake, since it is known to deplete calcium. I needed at least one cup in the morning. In the evening I had decaf coffee or herbal tea. I drank some diet sodas. And I tried very hard to increase my water intake.

Food Preparation

When I was at home and cooked, it was easy to stick to the rules. But since my husband and I no longer have any of our children living with us and we both work all day, we usually like to go out for dinner, alone, or with friends. This leads me to:

Strategies for Eating Out

1) *Eating out in my home town.* My first meal at a New York restaurant filled me with what I had begun to call prednisone angst. I was unduly nervous and ridiculously embarrassed. After my husband assured me I'd find things to eat and, if not, we'd just go home, I agreed to attempt my first dinner outside our own kitchen. The menu listed plenty of salads and vegetables and proteins, but all of them came with sauces, and even if I requested sauce on the side, what about the salt?

When it was my turn to order, I practically hyperventilated. "I'll have a house salad, please," I began, sounding meek and mousy, "but no dressing. I'd like olive oil and lemon wedges on the side. And then is it possible to have a plain grilled piece of salmon, or any kind of fish, with some steamed vegetables, no salt, and no butter?"

The waiter was silent. He looked confused.

"It's a medical thing," I quickly explain. "I'm sorry it's so complicated, but I can't have salt or . . ."

My husband's calming hand reached for mine just as the waiter said, "Sure, no problem."

I was practically in tears. I felt pathetic. Humiliated. My lower lip quivered. My husband squeezed my hand. "No one," he says, "needs to know the why of your requests." He told me not to apologize, just to ask directly for what I want. It took several more dinners out for me to stop feeling anxious as menus were handed around and to quit sounding apologetic when I ordered. I discovered that when I asked for what I wanted with an assertive rather than tentative tone I began to gain control over my angst. Being on prednisone, I decided, means never having to say you're sorry about special food requests.

I had no problem in ordering what I needed in two types of restaurants: really good restaurants and really simple coffee shops. Good restaurants were always accommodating, and in the average New York coffee shop no salt is used in food preparation anyhow. However, ethnic restaurants were out of bounds, except for those few Chinese restaurants that offered "diet dishes" such as plain steamed chicken with snow peas, and steamed rice. Most ethnic restaurants salt or marinate their food before preparation. I love Indian food and that was off-limits, as were almost all the hot and spicy places in town.

2) *Eating out on the road . . . in the United States.* My first trip out of town (see chapter 5) was to Houston, Texas, and on to

Oberlin and Bowling Green, Ohio. I had ordered a low-sodium meal for my flight, in advance; but nonetheless, I boarded the plane armed with rice cakes, a few apples, some salt-free sunflower seeds, and a small bottle of salt-free lemon pepper seasoning. The low-sodium meal was quite nice, if tiny. Once I arrived in Houston, I had no trouble ordering a dinner that was so good it needed none of my salt-free seasoning. The next morning at breakfast, I was surprised that the egg white omelette had reached the Deep South and was available at the hotel coffee shop. In Ohio, however, I had a greater challenge. In Oberlin I managed, after much negotiation, to get a salt-free meal. But in Bowling Green, no such luck. I arrived starving, needing lunch, and I had little time before my rehearsal. None of the places I tried could accommodate me. I had rented a car, and so I tooled around until I found a large grocery store. I stocked up on yogurts and fruits and found a really nice salad bar from which I could find exactly what I needed. I even found salt-free rice cakes. And after the concert someone suggested a restaurant that happily complied with my special requests.

3) *Eating out in Europe*. Prague! I was absolutely thrilled to have a concert there. But I had visited Czechoslovakia a few years earlier. Then all the food was gray and heaped with larded sauces and there were no fresh vegetables or fruits. Oh well, I decided. I'd take what salt-free foods I could and hope for the best. I remembered being on tour in Europe some years earlier with an orchestra from what was then called the Eastern Bloc. The musicians ate, as they put it, "out of their suitcases." In order to save money they packed canned tuna, canned beans, et cetera. And as I piled some tins of no-salt-added sardines as well as bags of rice cakes and other salt-free goodies, I couldn't help seeing the irony of being the indulged American who would be eating out of her suitcase.

The low-sodium meal I had ordered for my flight to the Czech

Republic was practically inedible. I hoped this was no indication of things to come. I landed in Prague excited about making music but resigned to starvation. I could not have been more wrong. Prague is not only elegant and cosmopolitan these days, filled with stands of fresh produce, but it offers some exquisite international eateries. I also happened to stay at one of the loveliest hotels I've ever been at, the Hoffmeister, run by a spirited young couple of that name, whose French chef was only too happy, so it was written on the menus, "to comply with your dietary needs." It was a far cry from Bowling Green, and I ate like a salt-free queen.

4) *Eating out at a dinner party.* Few of our friends have time to prepare dinner parties these days. We always seem to meet at restaurants. But when David and I were asked to someone's home for dinner, my prednisone angst kicked in. I called our hosts—good friends—and told them I had this restricted diet and offered to bring my own food. No no, they responded, they would be happy to make special food for me. But as I reeled off the list of my dietary no-nos I could almost see their eyeballs roll. Nonetheless, they were insistent on cooking for me, and they did. But I felt I had imposed on them, and that made me uncomfortable. In the future, I did not ask. I told the hosts I was bringing my own food. And from then on, I was a happier, more secure guest.

A Summary of Strategies for Eating Out

1) Avoid ethnic restaurants.
2) Do not be embarrassed to ask a waiter for whatever you need. And don't apologize.
3) Bring your own salt-free condiments.
4) Travel with some salt-free snacks. For plane trips, order low-sodium meals in advance.

5) BYOF. When you are invited to a dinner party, Bring Your Own Food.

6) Remember that your dietary restrictions are not arbitrary deprivations. By crafting a regime for yourself, you are not only beating the bloat. You are also taking some responsibility in your own recovery.

Exercise

Julie Some doctors tell patients on steroids that they can't do sports or heavy exercise, with the result that their patients become couch potatoes, aggravating the weight gain and muscle weakness that accompany treatment with this medicine. In fact, it is extremely important to prescribe exercise consistent with each patient's ability and conditioning. In my sister's case, had she not exercised, she'd have lost muscle strength and bone mass. She might also have gained a good deal of weight. Eugenia devised low-impact aerobic exercises that kept her in shape.

Eugenia I knew exercise was important during prednisone therapy not only to keep my weight down, but also to prevent bone loss. At first I felt too weak and worried to do more than easy morning stretches. But soon I was strong enough to take long strolls and then to go back to walking on the treadmill. Because of a back problem, jogging is out for me. But I've been a "power walker" for years. It seems to kick-start my metabolism, wake me up. Being able to roll out of bed in the morning and hit the treadmill gives me a sense of self-control and well-being. During my prednisone therapy, when my moods were in constant flux, exercise was more important than ever. It seemed to lift my spirits; it allowed me to start the day feeling upbeat. Although I was not always strong enough to walk as long or as fast as I had before the treatment, I was able to use the tread-mill with some consistency. At first I pushed myself, and then I paid for overdoing it with overwhelming fatigue later in the day. Then I learned to listen to my body and stop when I needed to without feeling that I had wimped out. "Go for the burn" is not a helpful slogan when you're slogging through a long course of prednisone.

I realize how fortunate I was to have been able to exercise at all during my illness. I knew that some patients on long-term prednisone therapy are too sick to be physically active. Yet despite my rigorous diet and exercise, I began to notice changes in my body. Although I had actually lost weight, there was nonetheless some odd shifting going on. There seemed to be a pronounced puffiness in my lower back, just above my kidneys. At first I thought it was water retention. But my doctor said it was not edema; it was the cushingoid effect, a weight gain around the trunk of the body. In my case, the gain was very slight. "It's hardly noticeable," I was told. But I noticed it. And even though I was assured it would fade eventually some months after I stopped prednisone, I worried that it would get worse. What if, after all my efforts, I ended up with a prednisone-induced middle age spread anyhow? Part of me wanted to give in, throw the diet to the winds, stop exercising. But then I realized that without all my hard work and self-control I probably would have really blown up. I decided to continue to count my calories . . . and my blessings. I was recovering, breathing easily, feeling well. I was truly lucky.

7

Coping
with Other
Side Effects

Julie *This chapter discusses a wide variety of additional side effects that can occur when you are on glucocorticoid therapy and will provide some strategies to help you deal with them. The chapter also contains some suggestions for what to do when it appears to you that your side effects are so marked that you wonder whether some other medical strategy should be indicated.*

The lists of side effects caused by steroids *are* long and intimidating. Most patients find reading them frightening and depressing. However, in writing this book we want to make the reader aware of risks as well as benefits when steroid therapy is required. Furthermore, advance knowledge makes it possible to do some prevention or, at least, to anticipate possible problems. It is *unlikely* that you will get all—or even a majority of—these side effects.

The accompanying box (page 64) details various categories of adverse reactions to steroid therapy. One of the more common manifestations of steroid side effects is that patients can become "cushingoid": they develop a round face, a ruddy complexion, thickening around the midriff and upper back. The term is derived from Cushing's disease, named after Dr. Harvey Cushing, who noted the same changes in body contour in patients with tumors that stimulated their own adrenals to make too much steroids. Years later, after steroid treatment was introduced, the term *cushingoid* was coined to describe the physical changes noted above that occurred in patients who were taking high-dose steroids.

Endocrine (Glandular) and Metabolic Changes

Many generalized changes in body metabolism occur when a person takes steroids. For most individuals, these changes are not profound. For others, the changes are marked. Depending on the tissue, steroids can lead to protein breakdown, especially in muscle, skin, fat, and lymphatic tissue; these effects are called catabolic. They make a person weaker. In the liver, steroids are called anabolic, meaning they lead to increase in production of fat and starch and in the capacity to make new sugar. These don't make you stronger, but they have a tendency to make you gain weight easily. Furthermore, steroids have a major effect on how the body handles sugars and may worsen diabetes or even induce it.

Skin and Hair Changes

Steroids can and often do cause many skin changes—thinning of the skin, stretch marks (striae), purple marks (purpura), and

---

Adverse Reactions to Glucocorticoid Therapy

Note: Most people do not develop these problems. In developing any particular side effect, the manifestation is usually mild.

Endocrine (Glandular) and Metabolic Changes

Change in body contour, with fat deposits on trunk, on the cheeks (moon facies), over the back of the neck (buffalo hump), around the neck (collar), yet sparing of the arms and legs

High blood sugar (steroid diabetes)

Increase in blood fat (hyperlipoproteinemia)

Negative balance of calcium, nitrogen, potassium (catabolic state)

Salt retention

Suppression of the adrenal glands (from the administered [exogenous] steroid)

Menstrual abnormalities

Impotence

Suppression of growth in children

Skin and Hair Changes

Facial redness (plethora)
Thin, fragile skin
Bruising
Stretch marks (violaceous striae)
Acne
Slow wound healing
Thinning of scalp hair
Increased body hair

Eye Changes

Cataracts (posterior subcapsular cataracts)
Increased intraocular pressure (glaucoma)
Eyeball prominence (exophthalmos)

acne. They also produce a redness of the cheeks (plethora) and increased sweating, as well as slow healing. In addition, steroids can cause an increase in body hair. Furthermore, thinning of scalp hair may take place.

All of this seems, at first, surprising, since steroids are useful

Adverse Reactions to Glucocorticoid Therapy, cont.

Muscle and Bone (Musculoskeletal) Changes

Weak muscles (myopathy)
Osteoporosis (bone structural weakening and thinning with possible compression fractures, spontaneous fractures)
Osteonecrosis of bone ends (noninfectious loss of blood supply to the ends of bone, with subsequent arthritic problems)

Gastrointestinal (GI) Side Effects

Gastritis
Peptic ulcer
Thrush
Pancreatitis

Cardiovascular Changes

Hypertension
Congestive heart failure (in predisposed patients)

Mood/Neuropsychiatric Changes

Alterations in mood
Psychosis
Convulsions
Pseudotumor cerebri (benign intracranial hypertension)

Infectious/Immune Changes

Increased susceptibility to infections
Suppression of immune responses (decreased inflammatory response; suppression of delayed hypersensitivity)
Change in the white blood cell population, with increase in some cells (neutrophils) and decrease in others (lymphocytes and monocytes)

for a wide variety of skin conditions. Nonetheless, the broad array of skin changes induced by steroids can be problematic.

Skin Changes

Thinning of the skin. Long-term use of steroids can result in a direct inhibition of skin fibroblast proliferation and affect synthesis of skin collagen, a supporting matrix structure. This means that your skin becomes thin, bruises easily, and does not heal well. Minimal trauma can cause marked damage, with appearance of big bruises. People on steroids should be very careful to keep their skin clean, protected, and intact.

The age and sex of the individual patient affects the degree of thinning and atrophy that occurs in the skin. In general, men have thicker skin than women, so that men usually experience fewer skin problems. In contrast, younger people have thicker skin than older individuals, and the presence of both male and female sex hormones in the young helps preserve skin thickness. Postmenopausal women are particularly at risk for developing thin, bruisable, atrophied skin.

Plethora. Steroids lead to loss of subcutaneous tissue, which causes redness of the face (plethora) because with less tissue under the primary layers of skin, the circulation is close to the surface. Of course, people on prednisone can have facial redness for other reasons, including sunburn, other medical conditions, or medications besides prednisone. Thus, before facial flushing is ascribed to steroids other reasons should be explored.

Stretch marks—striae. Stretch marks, or striae, can occur in people who take high-dose steroids. These stretch marks are particularly unsightly, wide (often over one centimeter in diameter), purplish (violaceous) striped areas that appear mainly on the abdomen but can also occur on the lower back, hips, buttocks, upper thighs, breasts, and upper arms. Steroid striae are different from those seen during normal pregnancy or with rapid weight gain, in which the stretch marks are thinner and pinkish while they develop and later become even thinner and silvery as they heal. In contrast, steroid stretch marks are big, wide, and unsightly. Luckily, not everyone gets steroid stretch marks. However, once stretch marks appear, they leave permanent scars. After a time, steroid stretch marks fade and become less noticeable, but even with treatment, they don't go away.

Why do stretch marks occur? There are areas of the dermis that have decreased supporting structure and thinning, but these thinned areas are not uniform. So some patchy loss of skin elasticity occurs, along with weakening of the underlying supporting tissue. This, along with weight gain, makes something "give," leaving stretch marks.

In recent years, various treatments have been tried to reduce stretch marks, but none has been proved to be particularly effective. Some recommendations are as follows:

- Avoid sunburn, especially on stretch marks. Use at least level 15 or higher of a sunscreen lotion.
- Try rubbing vitamin E oil into the skin once or twice a day. You can purchase vitamin E oil at most health food stores.
- Use water/oil massage cream. This has been tried for treating stretch marks in pregnancy and people are enthusiastic about the results, and it may help prevent or lessen steroid stretch marks.
- Use topical tretinoin, 0.025 percent cream, daily, for six or more months. Topical treatment with tretinoin has been described as improving stretch marks after pregnancy. While stretch marks from steroids are generally more pronounced than those that occur in pregnancy, the tretinoin may help.
- Laser treatment of stretch marks is experimental at this time yet very promising. In the future this may be a useful and effective approach.

Steroid acne.   Steroid acne, characterized by pimples and raised areas without pus, is typical. Pimples form at the base of hair follicles and skin pores. Changes in how quickly the components of those hair follicles and pores "turn over" may contribute to steroid acne. Teenagers will find steroid acne very distressing, and early referral to a dermatologist is recommended. Here are some suggestions that may help prevent or improve steroid acne:

- Be sure to keep the skin as clean as possible, avoiding oily creams that can seal off pores.
- Use topical antiacne medications.
- Consider taking antibiotics, being sure that those chosen will not interact with steroids.

Acanthosis nigricans.   A skin finding called *acanthosis nigricans* can occur when a patient is on steroids. This is a dark, soft, velvety change in the skin in areas that rub together, such as under the arm, in the groin, around the belt line, and at the bra line. The skin in such areas may not only be velvety but have small foldings and little skin tags (papillae). *Acanthosis nigricans* is thought to be due to a change in the supporting matrix of the skin.

Hair Changes

Several changes in hair can occur when a patient is on steroids. It is especially common to develop downy hairs on the forehead or upper cheeks. These hairs are usually fine and light in pigment and thus not cosmetically unsightly. However, an increase in the amount of pigmented, differentiated hairs can also occur in these areas, causing much distress.

What can you do if you develop an increase in facial hair?

- Use chemical epilation, with brands such as Surgicreme, which is hypoallergenic. This method works well for a moderate increase in hair. It is likely better than plucking or waxing. However, since the skin may be particularly sensitive, it is crucial to be sure that any residue of the hair removal cream is well rinsed from the skin after treatment. Otherwise an unpleasant chemical burn or skin rash is likely to occur.

- Avoid plucking and waxing, since your skin is likely to be very sensitive and to bruise easily.
- Consider shaving in some areas, but be careful not to nick the skin. Electric razors may be preferable to razors with blades.
- For marked increase in facial hair, consider electrolysis, being sure that meticulous local care and topical antibiotics are used to avoid infection.

Scalp hair changes.   Most people on prednisone notice little change in the hair on their heads. Some individuals notice a change in how curly their hair is. Others notice that their hair may become thin. This is partly due to conversion of administered steroid to androgens. If this occurs, it makes sense to consult a hair loss center, where they are skilled at making hair look thicker. In general, shorter hair has less tendency to fall out.

You may wonder why steroids cause so many skin side effects when topical or oral steroids are often used to treat skin conditions. The skin side effects of *long-term*, high-dose steroids seem paradoxical. Simply stated, the skin conditions that respond to steroids do so because inflammation is decreased by the medication. However, the effects of high-dose steroids on the skin and the layers of tissue beneath lead to structural changes that ultimately can damage the skin.

Gastrointestinal (GI) Side Effects

Several GI side effects are well recognized, but this does not mean you will suffer these complications. Most individuals experience only minor stomach discomfort and, possibly, thrush in their mouths. However, steroid-related intestinal complications can include gastritis, peptic ulcer (stomach ulcer), esophageal ulcers, GI fungal overgrowth (thrush), and pancreatitis (inflammation of the pancreas). The higher the dose and the longer an individual takes glucocorticoids, the more risk there is of GI side effects. It is also thought that the likelihood is somewhat greater if you already have GI problems such as stomach ulcers. The following paragraphs describe what you, in consultation with your doctor, can do to prevent GI side effects.

Stomach irritation and ulcer.   Steroid ulcers can be a possible complication with long-term steroid use, though the association has been controversial over the years. However, the association of steroids and gastric irritation or frank peptic ulcer is sufficiently well known that it may be wise to take some preemptive steps to prevent these unpleasant possibilities. This can be achieved by taking medications that will cut down stomach acid, block release of stomach acid, or coat the lining of the stomach. Thus, Tums or other antacids (which will have the additional benefit of increasing calcium intake, which may help osteoporosis) can be easy to take and helpful. It may also be worthwhile to take histamine H2 receptor antagonists (H2 blockers) such as cimetidine (Tagamet) or ranitidine (Zantac), which prevent release of acid from acid-secreting cells in your stomach lining. Prilosec may also prevent acid release. Another strategy is to use a medication that coats the lining of the stomach, such as bismuth (found in Pepto-Bismol) or sucralfate. While you can obtain these medications over-the-counter, it is advisable to discuss preventive treatment for stomach irritation with your doctor, since these medications could affect the effectiveness of other medicines you may be taking or may need.

Thrush. Oral thrush, a whitish coating in your mouth and tongue due to candida, a fungus, can easily occur if you are on high-dose steroids. Babies often get thrush in their mouths and diaper areas, and people taking glucocorticoids can get oral thrush too. Most of the time, this problem is simply an annoyance, though occasionally, oral thrush can be widespread, with involvement of the esophagus and other parts of the GI tract. The likelihood of such severe thrush can be prevented by using an antifungal mouthwash such as nystatin in a swish-and-swallow routine, several times per day to help prevent or control this problem. You should not embark on using nystatin on your own but should ask your health-care team about using nystatin mouthwash.

Muscle Changes

Both muscle wasting and muscle pain may occur while you are on steroids. Muscle becomes weaker, and may cause you a feeling of general weakness. As a result it is best to do new exercises slowly, in order to prevent muscle injury. Yet, staying active is crucial in order to prevent muscle atrophy.

Steroids should be used with caution in patients with heart conditions, as the heart muscle may be susceptible to damage.

Bone Changes

Steroids decrease bone density and strength and can lead to what is called osteoporosis. Steroids cause osteoporosis by several mechanisms. Bone is a dynamic tissue in which there is constantly a balance of new bone forming and older bone naturally remodeling itself (resorption). Steroids decrease bone formation but increase bone resorption, which leads to an overall decrease in bone density. This means your bones can be weakened by steroids. Furthermore, steroids inhibit intestinal calcium absorption and increase calcium excretion through the kidneys. So, less calcium is available to be laid down in bone. Since calcium is necessary for strong bones, it can be seen that steroids can place the body into a calcium-debt state. Steroids also inhibit adrenal synthesis of estrogen precursors, so that less active estrogen is available. This hormonal loss can increase the tendency to osteoporosis in both males and females.

Some people are more prone to develop bone problems while on steroids than others. Postmenopausal women are at risk for osteoporosis whether or not they are taking steroids. The addition of steroids may aggravate bone loss for such women. Children with growing bones are also at risk. Children need to be in positive calcium balance in order to grow, and steroids may place them into negative calcium balance.

Fortunately, much can be done to anticipate and lessen steroid-induced bone problems. For example, osteoporosis often can be prevented or minimized by increasing calcium in the diet or by providing calcium pills. Tums, which consist of calcium carbonate, are an effective calcium source that can also help prevent stomach ulcers. Steroids and antacids should not be taken simultaneously during the day, because they can bind to each other, so that steroids become less effective.

If osteoporosis is present when a course of steroids starts or develops during steroid treatment, then increased calcium intake, together with low-dose estrogen, will be helpful for postmenopausal women. Other therapy, such as calcitonin and vitamin D supplements, and biphosphonates may be helpful.

You should discuss your risks (or your child's risks) for osteoporosis with your doctor when the decision to start steroids is made. It is important for you to ask whether special precautions are indicated.

Eye Changes

Two types of eye problems can occur from being on high-dose steroids—cataracts and glaucoma. Fortunately, both of these complications are unusual and, furthermore, don't usually interfere with vision. Yet these are serious complications for which you should be monitored if on long-term steroids.

Cataracts.   Cataracts, opacities in the crystalline lens of the eye, can be brought on by steroids, with an incidence related to both the dose and duration of steroid treatment. How and why do these opacities form? What can you do, if anything, to prevent them? Do they ever go away on their own?

Cataracts occur in many circumstances. Cataracts can be part of normal aging, can be congenital, or can occur after eye injury, and treatment usually is removal and placement of an artificial lens. Cataract operations are now done in outpatient settings with excellent results. However, you are not likely to need surgery for steroid cataracts, even in the unlikely event that these cataracts develop in your eyes. Steroid cataracts are small and structurally different from other types of cataracts and usually don't interfere with vision.

Why do steroid cataracts occur? Steroids appear to be able to attach (bind) to proteins that make up the lens. Specifically, steroids bind to the amino acid lysine, forming a new steroid-protein compound that is opaque. This kind of compound is unique to steroid-induced cataracts and is not seen in other human cataracts.

Can you do anything to prevent steroid cataracts? No, you

probably cannot do anything to prevent yourself from forming steroid cataracts. The chance you'll get them is small. As mentioned above, steroid cataracts do not usually interfere with visual acuity but may require attention if they become large. You probably wouldn't even know that you've formed a steroid cataract. For this reason, you should have an ophthalmologic exam before or at the time of initiating high-dose steroid therapy. And you should have subsequent annual examinations.

Do these cataracts ever go away on their own? Yes, there are reports that steroid cataracts go away after a time; this is, however, the exception, not the rule. How and why the steroid cataracts may go away is just as mysterious as how they form.

Glaucoma. Steroids can raise the pressure inside the eye (this pressure is called intraocular pressure). Elevated intraocular pressure is known as glaucoma. If the rise in intraocular pressure is severe, it can lead to loss of visual acuity or even blindness. For this reason, an opthalomologist should check your intraocular pressure and follow it while you are on glucocorticoid therapy.

Increased intraocular pressure can be treated with medication, so it is very important to know whether you are developing this condition.

Mood/Neuropsychiatric Changes

This issue is very important when you are on steroids and may affect the success of your treatment. See chapter 5 for a detailed discussion of the issue.

Infectious/Immune Changes

Steroids can help the body fight certain infections, especially when the adrenals are not functioning well. At the same time, steroids can and do render people *more* susceptible to certain infections. Why is this? Partly because the effects depend on the dose. If someone needs a dose just high enough to balance his or her adrenal insufficiency, then the amount of steroids given will allow the body to respond appropriately to stress, even stress from severe infection. Once someone is on high doses for a month or more, however, the frequency of secondary infections will increase. At that point the body's ability to respond and fend off the usual skin and soft tissue infections and other infections, like urinary infections, pneumonia, and the like, is decreased. In other words, high-dose steroids compromise the body's ability to fight off certain infections.

Immune Response

Steroid therapy is sometimes intentionally used to lower immune reactivity. That is why, for example, steroids are helpful in treating autoimmune diseases (conditions such as lupus, in which the body "attacks" itself). They also help prevent transplant rejection. While these are important positive effects, steroids also can suppress the immune response in certain ways that may mask other problems. For instance, steroids can prevent assessment of skin tests for tuberculosis (tine tests or PPDs). Thus a person taking steroids may not react to the skin test even if he or she has TB, because the medication suppresses his or her response. For this very reason, whenever possible, it is of great importance to do TB skin testing *before* steroids are begun. Then, if there is a positive skin test, the potential need for treatment can be considered prior to initiation of the steroid therapy.

Susceptibility to Infection

Most people taking steroids do not need to worry about the increased chance of getting infections. Steroids don't make it more likely that you will catch bad colds. However, there are several infections that can be far more dangerous to a person on steroids—chickenpox (varicella) and other herpes viruses. Thus, before you start steroids, you should be sure to tell your doctor whether you (or your family member) have had chickenpox. If you are unsure or don't recall if you have had chickenpox, a blood test called a varicella (chickenpox) titer should be obtained. Chickenpox can be particularly severe in individuals taking high-dose steroids, and fatalities can occur. While there is now a vaccine (Varivax) against chickenpox, you cannot be immunized with it while you are on high-dose steroids. If you are susceptible to chickenpox (varicella) and you are exposed, you should get a shot of a special gamma globulin (varicella immune globulin, or V-ZIG) within seventy-two hours. If, in spite of being given gamma globulin, chickenpox develops, antiviral medicine such as acyclovir or ganciclivir can be lifesaving. It is important to discuss the varicella issue with your doctor before you start steroid treatment.

Anyone can develop shingles, also called herpes zoster, once he or she has had chickenpox, because the herpes zoster virus stays in your body. If you are on steroids, you are more prone to develop shingles than other people. Again, if shingles develops, the use of antiviral medications like acyclovir or ganciclivir will shorten the course of this painful illness.

Hypertension

The blood pressure in many, if not most, patients on long-term steroids increases compared to pre-treatment blood pressure.

Yet, actual high blood pressure is not present in that many patients. Some people, however, have or develop high blood pressure that requires medication for the duration of their steroid
therapy.

You should have your blood pressure measured before you
start steroids, and blood pressure should be checked at your
follow-up visits. If your blood pressure rises to a hypertensive
level, it should be treated while you need to be on the steroids.

Should you develop high blood pressure, it usually causes no
symptoms but will be detected at checkups. The high blood pressure that accompanies steroid use may respond to diuretic medication. However, other blood pressure medications besides
diuretic may be needed.

You can help to prevent high blood pressure by sticking to a
no-added-salt diet, by reducing stress as much as possible, and
by exercising.

Avascular Necrosis (Osteonecrosis)

In very rare instances blood supply to the bone ends becomes
compromised in patients taking high-dose steroids for long periods of time, causing these segments of bone to die off (necrose).
The upper ends (heads) of the femur (thigh bone) or humerus
(upper arm bone) are most often affected. Osteonecrosis is
painful and ultimately can cause arthritic problems. Fortunately,
this problem is infrequent and becoming less so with the present trend to use lower doses of steroids than was previously the
case.

8

Special Situations: Glucocorticoid Treatment in the Very Young and the Very Old

Julie *Sometimes the patient receiving glucocorticoids is a child or an elderly person. Both the young and the old have specific needs that must be considered by the health-care team and the family. This chapter provides some suggestions for five groups of patients: infants, young children, teenagers, elderly patients, and developmentally retarded patients.*

Infants and Glucocorticoid Therapy

There are few situations in which an infant needs long-term steroids. Undoubtedly, if you have a baby who is being given steroids, the reasons have already been discussed with you at length. Under these rare circumstances, it is important to be sure you understand the reasons for this therapy and have the baby monitored closely during the course of the medicine.

A large proportion of infants taking glucocorticoids need the medicine for replacement therapy—in order to replace steroids that the body is not making at all (adrenal insufficiency) or to replace steroids that are a different compound from normal and causing problems (most commonly, congenital adrenal hyperplasia). An infant with any of these conditions must be followed by a pediatric endocrinologist, a specialist in glandular diseases for children, who will help you monitor the baby for the important therapeutic effects of steroids in these conditions and will help you in handling any side effects. In fact, if your baby is on steroids for replacement therapy, you probably already have an endocrinologist. Steroids in replacement doses are unlikely to cause extra side effects, simply because the dose is intended to replace the steroids that the adrenal glands would be making under normal circumstances.

Occasionally an infant may need glucocorticoids to treat a specific condition, and the doses are likely higher than with replacement therapy. If so, the side effects that have been mentioned elsewhere in this book can occur, but the manifestations can vary in a baby. During the first year of life, babies triple their birthweight and grow many inches. Nutrition and metabolic balance are crucial to the future development of any human being. Thus I would recommend that any baby who needs to be on steroids be watched very closely.

Giving your baby any medicine can be tough, since medicines taste, well, like medicine. You should obtain an accurate measuring spoon or dosage tube from your pediatrician or at a pharmacy or food store. These are very helpful, because they are designed to be accurate and to be less likely to spill before the medicine is taken. Steroids do come in suspension form for babies and young children, but these preparations are rather bitter. Alternatively, steroid pills can be crushed up and put into applesauce. You can mix steroids in foods such as cereal, jam, applesauce, or pudding. Or you can mix the medicine with formula or other liquid. In this case, it is important to be sure the baby takes the whole dose, so that mixing it into a large amount of formula is not wise. A better strategy is to mix the medicine with an ounce or two of formula or other liquid, and when the baby has had that small amount switch to regular formula. If the baby is taking several medicines, then it is important that you know which is to be given when.

Diet needs to be appropriate for your baby's age. A very young baby should simply be on breast milk or formula, and diet should not vary. Breast milk tends to be very low in sodium, and most formulas in the United States are quite low in sodium content. It is worth checking with your doctor to be sure that the lowest possible salt formula is used. If the baby is ravenously hungry on steroids, you should watch how much formula and baby food he or she consumes, so that overfeeding does not get out of hand. If the baby is a bit older and if solid foods have been introduced, be sure that a very hungry baby takes in relatively lower calorie foods. A baby should be gaining weight and growing, so you should use the following guidelines about weight gain:

Age	Calories/Day	Total Calories	Daily Weight Gain
1–6m	Kg x 108	520–780	15–30 gm/day ($\frac{1}{2}$–1 ounce)
6–12m	Kg x 98	680–1020	10–15 gm/day ($\frac{1}{4}$–$\frac{1}{2}$ ounce)

Source: Stallings VA. *Nutrition for Normal Infants, Children and Adolescents.* In Burg F., Ingelfinger J., Wald E., Eds. *Current Pediatric Therapy* 14, W. B. Saunders Co., Phila., 1993, p. 2.

Looking at this table, you'll see that a young baby will gain between 1/4 pound and 1/2 pound in about 8 days, while an older baby gains that amount in about 2 weeks. So a baby gaining a pound in a week would be unusual. If your baby is gaining very rapidly, you might want to think of the calorie content of some baby foods:

Food	Calories per 3–ounce serving
Breast milk or formula	20 calories/oz (3 oz = 60 calories)
Baby cereal with formula	110
Baby cereal with water	50
Baby cereal in jars	55–70
Vegetables	25–70
Fruits and juices	40–80
Meats	90–135
Whole cow's milk	19 calories/oz
2% cow's milk	15 calories/oz
Skim milk	10 calories/oz

Thus this table tells you that some foods have more calories than other foods. For an older infant or toddler, using cereal without milk or with skim milk can be helpful.

Source: *Current Pediatric Therapy* 14, p. 3.

If your baby is gaining a huge amount of weight on steroids, then seeing a nutritionist or talking at length with your pediatrician or his or her staff about how to control the problem can be very important. In fact, seeing a nutritionist at the start of steroid therapy can be helpful. Remember, your baby *should* be gaining weight, but not to the point of becoming obese, as this can affect blood pressure and can even delay the baby's mobility and acquisition of large motor skills such as creeping and walking.

The same side effects that occur in older patients can occur in babies on steroids. However, the side effects may be harder to detect and harder to manage. A few aspects of the side effects that are different in a baby are worth noting. In reading about various problems you should remember that babies can't tell you what is wrong. Symptoms and signs of illness are quite nonspecific.

Hypertension.   Most babies taking steroids do have some increase in blood pressure after a few weeks. Most don't become hypertensive, but *markedly* high blood pressure is a side effect that may require medication. The hard thing about assessing blood pressure in a baby is measuring it. Despite blood pressure machines, measuring blood pressure accurately in a wriggly and/or irritable baby can be almost impossible. Blood pressure done while the baby is napping is likely to be more accurate than if he or she is awake and irritable. You should remember that blood pressure levels in babies are very much lower than those in older individuals, so that levels that would be totally normal for a parent are "sky-high" for a baby.

Gastrointestinal side effects.   Babies can't tell you if they have gastric or duodenal irritation. They may cry or act irritable. The baby should be placed preemptively on antacids and/or acid-lowering medications. You can assume that a baby on high-dose steroids may be at risk for oral and generalized thrush, and preemptively the baby should be on anti-thrush medication such as nystatin.

Children and Glucocorticoid Therapy

Children are normally growing and developing on a daily and monthly basis. Because steroids affect the body profoundly, steroid therapy presents particular problems for the child and family.

While the short-term use of high-dose steroids in a child does not usually pose a serious problem, it is important to watch several things that can lead to long-term difficulties. If a child is going to be on high-dose steroids for a prolonged period of time, then it is even more important to try to prevent problems. The following discussion points out some difficulties and how to minimize problems related to them.

Telling Your Child about Steroids

Talk to your child about the medicine in an age-appropriate way. A very young child really cannot discuss the use of the medicine and the whys and wherefores. A school-age child can talk about the medicine with you and with the doctor.

Taking the Medicine

Most children take steroids without complaint, but some really don't like the taste of the medicine. In that case, putting the medicine into foods can be helpful as long as it is not put into large portions where it may get "lost." Still other children are old enough to understand that they don't like how they *feel* on steroids and that weight gain is due to the medicine. If they balk at taking the medicine, then working out a system with positive reinforcement for sticking to the regimen will be critical.

Diet

A child may become voracious while receiving steroid therapy, gaining a great deal of weight if not supervised. A young child has little motivation, in general, for thinking about how he or she looks. The child simply feels starved and will eat anything and everything in sight. Therefore, it is important for parents to be sure that there is healthful, low-calorie food around, not junk food. It is crucial to inform others involved who interact with the child about this issue. Otherwise, these people may feed the child indiscriminately. Here are some suggestions:

- Write out your child's diet on a piece of paper and make this available to relatives, to baby-sitters, to school and after-school programs, and to parents of friends at whose homes the child spends time. Explain that he or she has a particular tendency to gain weight right now on the medication. Also, provide a list of high-salt and low-salt foods, as well as particularly encouraged snacks.
- Send snacks with your child to school or to friends' houses.
- Make a system of sticker or star rewards for your child for snacking on the right foods.

Sports for the Child on Steroids

If a child is on high-dose steroids, most activities are still fine. Most kids will monitor their own activities. The best exercises to encourage are aerobic noncontact sports, but keeping the child active is more important than the type of sport. Sedentary children use up fewer calories and tend to get out of shape. Thus I actually recommend that children on steroids have some sort of activity prescription.

Steroids and Mood

Some children become very moody on steroids, posing problems at home, at school, and with friends. Anticipate this possibility and talk to your child's teachers, to the parents of friends, and to those involved in your child's life. Usually this is all that is needed. Some children, however, have more problems, leading to major school difficulties, as well as disruption of family life and interference with friendships. In this case, it may be helpful to seek counseling and even to consider medication for the mood swings, if no other course of action works.

Teenagers on Glucocorticoids

It is tough enough to be a teenager, but a teenager taking a medicine like prednisone in high doses is going to be very distressed about the side effects. Thus getting the teen to understand why the medicine is needed is essential. Depending on the reason for the medicine, the teen will be more or less likely to "comply" with the prescription plan. "Noncompliance," or not following the medication plan (or the medical plan in general), is more common in teenagers than in other patient age groups. If steroids are needed to treat a serious disease, noncompliance can be life-threatening.

R.'s Story

R. has a rare lung and kidney disease called Goodpasture syndrome. At the time this condition was diagnosed, she was a beautiful willowy fourteen-year-old who hoped for a modeling career. Then she had a lung hemorrhage and acute nephritis that brought her to the hospital, and a renal biopsy rapidly led to the diagnosis. This particular disease can result in kidney failure and/or death. The fortunate part of the story is that after R. received prompt therapy, not only with steroids, but with cyclophosphamide and plasma exchange, her nephritis began to quiet down. However, R. needed long-term steroids. She took them willingly at first, but she did not keep track of her diet in any way. She ate lots of salty and sugary foods, became hypertensive, and gained over forty pounds. She developed cushingoid appearance, as well as many striae, or stretch marks. She looked chubby, and certainly though still attractive, she did not look like a candidate for the cover of *Seventeen Magazine* any longer. She became angry and depressed. She missed several clinic visits and also started skipping school. She showed up in the emergency room threatening suicide. While talking helped R. see the lifesaving value of steroids in her situation, she really didn't "get" the gravity of the situation. She took her medication sporadically at best.

It took two years, several flare-ups of her illness with life-threatening lung hemorrhages, and a large effort to win her confidence and help her to understand on a deep level how important taking her medicine is. Luckily, R. didn't die, which she could have; but her lung disease progressed. Today, at age eighteen, she has her disease under control, on low-dose prednisone, and is again willowy. She usually takes her medication as prescribed and usually, but not always, comes to the clinic. She hopes that laser therapy might help get rid of the stretch marks, but she is taking her medicine.

What Can Be Done?

Since steroids are needed when prescribed, it is especially important that *time* be spent explaining in depth and language that the teen understands why the medicine is needed, what its side effects can be, and how these can best be handled. Preemptive counseling can be invaluable.

Steroids and the Elderly

An elderly person requiring steroids may already have several of the problems that can be initiated as side effects by steroids, including thinning of the bones (osteoporosis), muscle weakness, cataracts, glaucoma, high blood pressure, and skin changes. These conditions will be aggravated by steroids. For this reason, alternative therapy should be used if possible. If steroids are necessary, elderly patients should be monitored very closely.

Steroids and the Developmentally Retarded

If steroid therapy needs to be prescribed for a patient with developmental retardation, the situation is analogous to steroid use in infants and young children, except, if the patient is adult size, getting the medicine into him or her can be a challenge. Furthermore, a number of people with developmental retardation are likely to need other medications. It is very important to focus on the possibility of the interaction of steroids with other medications, as discussed in chapter 4.

9

Changing
Doctors

This chapter is about changing doctors: when to do it, how to do it, pros and cons, patient rights.

Eugenia   Six weeks into my treatment, I changed doctors. It was a gut decision, one that snuck up on me, ambushed me, and made me act quickly. This is how it happened:

The initial diagnosis of my disease was made by a lung expert who was an excellent doctor. He took time to explain my illness to me in detail and to talk about a planned cure. He was willing to consult with my sister and her colleagues in Boston. But he was very busy, and I often had to wait to see him far longer than any patient would have liked. What's more, his office was in a hospital clinic where the waiting room was hot, stuffy, and uncomfortable. During my examinations, his emphasis on the fact that I was "very sick" and that the disease was "very serious" made me more nervous than I already was. In retrospect, I realize that I should have tried to ask him more questions and to tell him how I was really feeling. But somehow his doom-and-gloom attitude scared me into silence. And so did the nurse who drew my weekly blood. She always had such difficulty hitting the veins that my arms were constantly bruised and sore. My discomfort with the entire situation dawned on me six weeks into my treatment. One day I arrived at the hospital for my appointment and took the elevator up to the lung clinic as usual, only to find the usual entrance closed off. A large skull and crossbones was posted across the door with this message printed beneath it: "Do not enter. Asbestos removal." I thought it was very funny, at first—asbestos, which can cause major pulmonary problems, on the lung floor! But then I was alarmed. And as I followed a different and labyrinthine route to the lung clinic, I began to notice that the hospital seemed less than sparkling clean. I already knew that it was understaffed and personnel were not friendly, but what's more, I realized that its location was not convenient to my apartment. I suddenly asked myself in case of an emergency, would I want to be admitted to this hospital? My answer was a resounding: "No!"

I talked to Julie about my concerns. She said that if I did not feel confident where I was, making a change would be perfectly valid. "Patients often switch doctors," she said, "and a reasonable doctor will be understanding and cooperative."

But to whom should I switch? Julie did not know any lung specialists in New York. She said she would check with her colleagues and get back to me. In the meantime, I happened to speak to a friend who turned out to be a fountain of information on medical treatments. "I've got files on every disorder in the book," she said. "And I've kept the most recent list from *New York Magazine* of the best doctors in New York. I'll fax you the lung page. . . ."

She did. I noted that the doctor I had been seeing was not on the list. But there were thirty-nine "best" names under "Pulmonology." How would I begin to narrow the numbers down? Each doctor's name was followed by his/her hospital affiliation and specialty. I noticed that there were four doctors who specialized in "interstitial lung disease." My illness fit that category. All four interstitial lung disease experts were connected to fine private hospitals. But I certainly did not want to see all four of them. How would I make a choice? Serendipity again: I bumped into another friend whose mother, it turned out, was also being treated for a lung disease.

"I'm looking for a new lung doctor myself," I said.

"Look no further," my friend told me. "Daniel Libby, New York Hospital. He's the one for you. He's a great doctor, and so caring, so compassionate. My mother loves him!"

I checked my notes. Daniel Libby was one of the four doctors on my list. I called Julie. I asked her if it seemed reasonable for me to go see a doctor on the basis of my friend's mother's enthusiasm, and because of his inclusion in *New York Magazine*'s list of best doctors.

"Those magazine lists are fairly reliable," Julie answered. "Dr. Libby is at New York Hospital. It's a fine place. But most important is that he sounds like a good guy. You have it on the authority of one of his patients that he's caring and empathic. Make an appointment with him."

Prednisone angst suddenly grabbed me. "But what do I tell the doctor I'm seeing now? What if he gets mad at me? And what if I don't like Dr. Libby? And my x-rays and CAT scans, where are they? You've got them. What if they're lost and . . ."

There ensued a rather edgy exchange over the lost x-rays (which Julie describes in chapter 5). After we both calmed down,

Julie offered me some diplomatic strategy. She suggested I tell the doctor I was currently seeing that I had decided to consult someone else for a second opinion. Given the nature of my illness and its projected long-term care, it would be perfectly reasonable for me to ask to see another doctor.

I braved what I feared would be the wrath of the gods. But my doctor was reasonable, if subdued, at the news that I wanted a "consultation." I'm sure he suspected that I was looking to make a change. But he was cooperative nonetheless.

My first appointment with Dr. Daniel Libby coincided with a recent glitch with my medication. I had been taking sixty milligrams of prednisone every other day, but a blood test had alarmed my doctor, who had prescribed that I now take fifty milligrams one day and ten the next. In the taxi to Dr. Libby's office, I was worried about that recent blood test and generally nervous about meeting a new doctor. Recommendations aside, how would I know how to make a judgment? I suddenly remembered the time that I needed a urologist and was sent to one I knew nothing about. I had called Julie. Neither she nor her colleagues had heard of this urologist. She advised me to make sure to ask what medical school the doctor had attended. If it sounded reputable, I could rest assured that he would be competent. But the urologist's office had been filled with art and he was so interesting that I completely forgot to question him until there I was, spread-eagled on his table. "By the way," I asked, "where did you go to med school?"

"Belgium," he answered. "I couldn't get into a medical school in the States."

That urologist turned out to be a terrific doctor, and the incident taught me that a doctor's worth cannot be measured by which school he or she attended. But nonetheless, approaching Dr. Libby's office, I reminded myself to scan his walls for a medical school certificate. I was jumpy and anxious, but as I entered a clean, efficient building near New York Hospital and took the elevator up to see Dr. Daniel Libby, pulmonologist, I began to calm down. His secretary was friendly. The waiting room was pleasant, and I did not have to sit there more than a few minutes before I was called in to meet the doctor. Daniel Libby was tall and attractive, with a most appealing smile. I liked him immediately. We spoke first in his office, where photos of his wife and three daughters hung over his desk. A happy family struck me as an excellent recommendation.

Dr. Libby had read the files that had been faxed to him. He had already looked at the x-rays and CAT scans that I had given to his secretary. He agreed with the diagnosis. But he asked me many questions, and I was struck by his concern for detail, his seeming interest. I felt so comfortable and relaxed in his presence that I forgot to check out the walls for a medical school certificate.

In the examining room, things were equally easy. He said he felt that since my infiltrates were fading and my lungs were almost clear, I really should be lowering my dosage of prednisone.

"But my eosinophils went up," I said. "My doctor said I can't lower the dosage until the blood count is better."

Dr. Libby smiled that smile of his. "I treat patients," he said, "not lab reports."

I was more than impressed. I was bowled over. "Will you be my doctor?" I blurted.

"If you're sure you really want to make a change," he answered as he scribbled something on a chart. "But how do you know so quickly you'd like to?"

"Because," I pointed out, "you're left-handed. So am I."

Laughter. It brightened my mood, brought back my confidence, made me feel optimistic and positive. And then when Dr. Libby's nurse, June, came in to take my blood and hit a vein bull's-eye, and it didn't hurt at all, I knew I was in the right place.

When I got home, I called my friend whose mother was also being treated by Dr. Libby to thank her for the recommendation. "He's handsome, and he's left-handed," I gushed. "And best of all," I added, as if it were a minor detail, "he says he can cure me."

I of course consulted with Julie. She advised me that the degree of comfort with and confidence in a doctor and his hospital was important for my recovery. "Go ahead," she said. "Make the change." And again, she helped me decide what to say to my (now) former doctor. I dreaded that phone call. But I took a deep, clear breath and just did it. To my relief, my announcement was greeted with kindness. "I understand," the doctor said, at the end of our conversation. "And I wish you the best."

Julie   Patients change doctors for various reasons. Doctors know this, and most of the time the decision to switch will not pose a problem, the doctor will be understanding, and the transition will be smooth. Sometimes, however, there can be miscommunication and misunderstanding.

As she described, Eugenia had a list of reasons for switching doctors:

- Her initial doctor was very busy, and the long waiting times were in a busy, uncomfortable, and possibly unhealthful environment.
- She felt that his emphasis was on how ill she was rather than on how well she might get.
- The ancillary staff seemed solemn and gloomy and, what's more, had some difficulty drawing Eugenia's blood.
- She didn't think she'd be confident if she had to be an inpatient in this doctor's hospital.

Could there have been other, unstated reasons? None of us like bad news. A patient may feel a need to switch doctors just to put distance between the trauma of learning about a serious problem and coping with getting well again. I call this the "shoot the messenger" syndrome, and it may have played a role in Eugenia's decision. It may be better to work things through with the first doctor if this is the main reason for switching. It can be hard to know whether the motivation for switching is because of the bad news *per se*. From the physician's viewpoint, it takes patience and understanding to discuss this issue with a patient. When possible, it can be rewarding for both the patient and the doctor to work through the pain and despair of learning about a tough diagnosis and to develop a strong patient-doctor alliance afterward. If the patient understands the diagnosis and its implications and wants to get well, then the subsequent treatment and course are much easier for all—even if the outcome may be unsatisfactory. So, as a doctor, I try to recognize how the patient feels about his or her diagnosis, so that I can spend appropriate time talking it through. Still, time constraints, attitudes, and circumstances conspire so that this is not always possible.

All in all, the reasons patients switch physicians are many. Doctors *expect* that some of their patients will change doctors in the course of treatment. In fact, in an era of changes in health-care insurance, switching doctors has become very common for bureaucratic and pragmatic reasons. Furthermore, getting a "second opinion" is important, and it is part of standard care for some diagnoses.

Sometimes patients switch from doctor to doctor very often, seemingly hoping that the next practitioner will "get it right." Almost invariably, the inveterate "doctor shopper" stays dissatisfied. All the effort of going from doctor to doctor leaves the patient with confusing information overload, a huge time expenditure, and big bills. "Doctor shopping" is unrewarding for all concerned, usually because there is no continuity and because few or none of the doctors consulted get to understand the underlying concerns of someone who is so frantic that he or she is consulting many individuals.

So when should you get a second opinion? When should you switch doctors? There are specific instances when this makes sense.

When Should You Get a Second Opinion?

If your symptoms are pronounced and your diagnosis unclear, you should have another doctor review your records and meet with you. While such a consultation may lead to more testing without diagnosis, exploring the issues with another doctor and getting the same answer may be reassuring. On the other hand, the second consultant may change the diagnosis.

If you have a definite diagnosis, but tests or treatment carry substantial risks, side effects, or cost, you should seek further information. A second opinion can be very helpful in confirming the benefits and risks of what is suggested.

When Should You Switch Doctors?

Sometimes patients switch doctors for "no good reason." The differences in style between patient and doctor could have been worked out if only the patient and/or the doctor and staff had made a minimal effort—or if the patient had calmed down. If you are thinking of switching, ask yourself: "Is this a communication problem or a problem of style I can work through?" Whatever the reasons, if *you* are not comfortable with your doctor, you should try to resolve the differences you may have and to get answers to questions that bother you.

Sometimes a patient will switch because another doctor has been so highly recommended by the patient's family, colleagues, or friends that being under the care of the "new" doctor seems like the only way to assure "getting the best," even though the "old" doctor is doing a fine job. Sometimes, however, there is the sense that the first doctor is not, in fact, doing a good-enough job.

You should switch doctors if and when you feel deeply uncomfortable with your doctor, the office staff, or the environment. This could mean that:

- You feel that the way your doctor handles discussions with you is not right for you.
- You feel that something was mishandled and you have lost confidence in your doctor.
- You are angry with your doctor and cannot get past this.

Switching Doctors Due to Circumstances You Can't Control

You may need to switch doctors

- If your health insurance provider changes, an increasingly common problem.
- If you are moving to a new locale.
- If your doctor is moving, leaving practice, or becomes ill and/or dies. (In the case of the doctor being no longer available, it may be most expeditious to switch to one of that doctor's partners, if possible.)

How to Switch Smoothly

Switching doctors should not be a clandestine event. You should be totally open with your first doctor about it. You must be sure that your records are transferred expeditiously. Here are simple steps:

- Discuss the switch with your doctor and the doctor's office staff, providing the name and address of the other practitioner. Your reasons for switching should be clearly and calmly stated.

- Ask both doctors to talk over your case together. Most doctors are glad to do this, and it is often helpful.
- Obtain your records in advance so that the new doctor can review them, prior to your first visit if possible. (You may wish to have the records sent, or you may wish to deliver them in person.)
- Make biopsy slides and actual x-rays available to the new doctor. It is best if he or she can review these directly, in addition to reviewing the interpretations (reports).
- Keep lines of communication open.
- Most states permit patients to see their records. It is often necessary, nonetheless, to make a formal request prior to such a review. Requirements will vary from state to state and hospital to hospital. Your doctor's office should be prepared to facilitate such a request.

10

Attitude:
A Personal
Attempt to Think
Positive

NOTE: *A patient on long-term medication will have ups and downs. This is a personal account.*

Eugenia Changing doctors was a turning point for me. I was now under the care of a lung specialist whose positive attitude was catching. He told me that my disease was serious but controllable and that I would slowly begin to reduce the amount of prednisone I was taking. He said I would get well and stay well. His optimism made me believe that I was on the road to recovery.

My experience taught me what a large part attitude plays in getting better. No matter what the illness, being hopeful about the outcome makes an enormous difference. During the first six weeks that I was on megadoses of prednisone, I felt weak, frightened, and helpless. Yes, I had taken some steps to try to minimize the side effects of the medication. Outwardly I was "doing well." But inside, I was an emotional jellyfish. It was one thing to know that my moods were being distorted by prednisone; it was another to reclaim my inner strength. Finding a new doctor, one who was upbeat and positive, seemed to set me on the path to regaining my confidence.

In order to help speed my own recovery, I decided it was time to treat myself well. I began by changing my attitude toward physical therapies. Before my illness, I had viewed body work—massage, shiatsu, chiropractic—as something of a self-indulgence. I now realized that the gifted practitioner offers something beyond pleasure and/or relief. Ira Lieberman, the chiropractor I had been seeing from time to time in New York, not only aligned my spine but also made me feel well adjusted on a deeper level. I decided to see him regularly, and his help was invaluable. In the past, I had also enjoyed occasional sessions with Arthur Wooten, a truly talented practitioner of traditional Japanese shiatsu. Similar to massage in that it helps relax tense and exhausted muscles, shiatsu is like acupuncture in its concept that there are pressure points (*haras* in Japanese) that, when stimulated, will release energy throughout the body. But Arthur Wooten is more than a mere manipulator of muscles and pressure points. He has healing hands, his very presence is restorative, and his insights about mind/body/emotion interactions provide guidance and direction. Seeing him regularly made me believe that despite my disease, I was reasonably fit.

Allowing myself the help of a chiropractor and a shiatsu practitioner reinforced positive thought. But I still experienced major mood swings, sudden jolts of nervousness, edginess, and sleeplessness. I had decided early on in my treatment that because my emotional instability was being caused by prednisone, I would simply tough it out through the treatment. In retrospect, I wish I had seen a psychotherapist. Friends and family provided encouragement, but a professional could have helped me ferret out which feelings were real and which were prompted by prednisone. Talking about my illness, my fears, and my anxieties in a therapeutic setting might have offered relief. Of course I see this with twenty-twenty hindsight. At the time, I was myopic about my emotional state. Although I was aware that my responses to normal everyday situations were unusual, I was unaware of just how peculiar I was behaving while on the medication. How strange was I? I decided, when I was finally off the medicine, to ask some people who have known me before, during, and after my siege with prednisone.

"How strange were you?" one kind friend responded. "You weren't strange. You were just not yourself."

"You were strange," my daughter Arianna disagreed. "You were *weird*, Ma, as in *wacko*."

How did my weirdness manifest itself? I decided, six weeks after I was completely finished with my medication, to ask the man who was, and is, my closest companion—my husband, David. We had not conducted any sort of "postmortem" on prednisone. Perhaps we had both feared a candid assessment of that siege. But when we sat down to talk about how "different" I had been during my treatment, our conversation turned out to be both honest and illuminating.

In my work as a television correspondent, I have conducted many interviews. In all of these interviews, I've noted that the formality of taping a conversation ironically leads to candor and intimacy. The camera tends to be a truth machine—under its scrutiny, there's nowhere to hide. So, on a hunch that David and I would speak more openly if our conversation were taped, I recorded the following exchange. Even though it was audio alone, I do think that David felt somehow free to speak his truth, and so did I.

Interview with David Seltzer

EZ: So what was I really like during those ten months?

DS: You were filled with fear, panic. There was no fun, no lightness of being. Your reactions to things were exaggerated. You were angry and confrontational. I had to measure and weigh the things I said to you because you were easily inflamed. I was going through some really bad times myself, financially for instance, and I would sense that it would send you into a state of alarm if I was worried about it, or about other things. You were very alone, very isolated; there was no consoling that you would accept. You saw any attempts to help you as being invasive or judgmental or hostile. Any time that I would suggest anything to you about your illness, you would shut me out of it really fast and tell me that it was your business and that you were handling it and then you would complain that you were alone with it. So I would say isolation was something you were feeling, or creating for yourself. It might have been just that you were afraid you were going to die and felt that you needed to not give away any modicum of control; and you may have felt that even listening to someone's opinion or accepting sympathy was in some way admitting that you were in need. I don't think you were just trying to be stoic. I don't know how much of that is your personality in a life-threatening situation, but I will tell you that when people close to me would ask, "How's Genie?" I would often respond, "Genie is nuts." And then I would explain that you were taking prednisone and you were not yourself and that I felt very much alone.

EZ: I'm sorry you felt alone.

DS: We both did.

EZ: You said I was "nuts." What did "nuts" mean to you?

DS: Nuts meant that you didn't have normal responses to things. I wish I could find specific incidents . . .

EZ: What about the time, early on in the treatment, when I was terrified about the physical changes I feared were in store for me, and I asked you to take photographs?

DS: Right. You worked yourself into a frantic state, thinking, I suppose, that you wanted to document your own deterioration, which is pretty extreme. Then you posed as starkly as you could and asked me to snap away, which I did, and then when you saw the photographs, you were insulted and enraged that I hadn't tried to make you look better, that you looked so terrible. You sensed that I was delighting in photographing you looking so terrible. So I thought that was kind of bizarre.

EZ: Did you think there was any difference when I changed doctors to someone who was more upbeat?

DS: No, I didn't. I sensed that you were with a doctor who was perhaps sugarcoating things, and that it wasn't, on a deep level, making you feel any more secure. I think you always felt that you were on the road to doom; and I thought that was possible too, because you seemed so convinced of it, and I didn't know as much as I should about the illness itself. My closest friend would say to me, "Call a doctor; make her go see somebody else; bone up on it so you can discuss it." And I said to him, "She does *not* want me to have anything to do with it; she does *not* want me to discuss it with her. Every time I try to discuss it with her I am slam-banged out of it." And I did ask you many times to seek other opinions, especially when you were unhappy with that first doctor. Then you did, but certainly not on my advice.

EZ: I remember taking your advice. Like the time I had that relapse when I was playing in a summer music festival in Maine and was back on really high doses of prednisone; you came up there, and I listened to everything you said.

DS: In Maine, you were a mess. But that was not as atypical as you think. You were a very helpless person throughout much of your treatment, but you rarely admitted it. It was like you weren't really inhabiting yourself. You were running on the idea of who you were for a lot of your prednisone months: "This is how Eugenia behaves, so I'll behave that way." You were still making all the moves and you looked like you, but being with you was not like being with you.

EZ: Am I back to myself now, six weeks off the medication?

DS: Yes, I think you are back to yourself, and I think it was almost instant when you came off the prednisone. You were very helpless in many ways but not wanting to admit it. That time I saw you in Maine you had completely given up on being able to help yourself, and so it was easy for me to take charge. But I think you were finally admitting that you felt like an invalid, psychologically. You felt like you couldn't cope, and that was one situation that finally baffled you, and it was a fairly simple situation: you were put in a bad hotel room. You know, it's something any of us could figure out right away. You should have said to yourself, "This isn't good enough; I'm going to look for somewhere else as soon as I'm through with rehearsal." But because someone had told you, "That's where you're staying," you had agreed to imprisonment. And you were like a kid when I took you out. I felt like I was rescuing one of my kids, which I've done on occasion, when something has rendered them completely helpless. And I took you out into the world and put you in a decent hotel. At that point, I had that same sense that you had now become a very helpless person.

EZ: Did you worry throughout my illness that I was becoming really unbalanced, and did you start to think that it was something you would have a lot of difficulty coping with?

DS: I was kind of treading water with your situation. It was difficult, and I didn't know if it was the prednisone or if you were simply becoming batty.

EZ: Well, that's the trick; that's the conundrum of this. You're told that on this medication you can have mood swings; you're told that you can have almost psychotic behavior. But at what point are you able to say to yourself, "This is the prednisone; this is not me"? I think that what it does is just exaggerate the oddness of one's personality. Maybe it extends the extremes of one's behavior. What do you think?

DS: That sounds right to me. It's like everything I see in you, and I'm sure you see many things in me, that you hope don't get any worse because they're just marginally tolerable faults . . .

EZ: Moi? I have faults?

DS: You began acting like you were in enemy territory, all the time. It was as if forces inside of you and outside of you were all conspiring to shut you down, and you were in a struggle. I appreciated the fact that you had something that could kill you; and I thought, as you thought, that this might *actually* be the thing that kills you.

EZ: What's odd is that with the prednisone, I knew my disease was getting better. It was that I had been told that it's not a *curable* disease, it's a *repressible,* disease and that without prednisone it *can* kill you. I think that was the anger, the feeling that I didn't want to be taking prednisone, but if I didn't, the opposite choice was unacceptable; so I felt angry that I had to be in that bind.

DS: I know that no matter what goes on in our lives you and I usually wake up feeling light and silly and have funny conversations in the morning, which is one of the things that I've always loved about our marriage and waking up with you, that I can be goofy in the morning and you're very receptive to it. I was once married to a woman who had a clinical depression. And when she opened her eyes in the morning, *it* was there; and that's the way you were when you were taking prednisone. There was no more funny stuff in the morning. Your eyes opened, and you quickly focused on all the problems of the day and of your life and of the relationships and of your sadness. You had lost your father not long before that, but his death was something that was haunting you during that time. You were

sad. And you know, worst of all? It was the look in your eye
and the tilt of your head. When people said, "How's Genie?"
and I said, "Genie's nuts," that's exactly what I thought of. You
would walk into a room with your head tilted and your eye-
brows cocked, and you looked crazy. And I knew that you were
completely uncomfortable with the encounter that was about
to occur, which might have been as threatening as, "Hello; how
was your day?"

EZ: I guess I was completely weirded out on the medication.

DS: And tremendously self-conscious. Very much talking to
yourself all the time, not out loud, but you were in an internal
dialogue all the time; and, as such, almost seemed well rehearsed
for whatever conversations we were going to have. But you
looked batty; that's all I can say. And I honestly believe that if
you ever take a mood-altering drug that does what prednisone
did, I'll know it before you ever open your mouth just by the
way you toss your head.

EZ: What's astonishing is that at the time I had no idea. I
thought there was something wrong with people around me; I
thought other people were acting odd.

DS: It was *you*. I could even hear it in your voice on the
phone . . . and I could tell when you weren't really having a conversation with me.

EZ: In retrospect are there any things you would advise people in a similar situation, being the companion of someone on
megadoses of prednisone, to do that could help?

DS: Had you been my child or my patient, I do believe I would
have sat with you, held your hand, and waited it out longer until
we could have shared what was going on with you; but I was
having my own reactions of feeling angry that I was left alone
by your illness too, because I was going through some stuff. We
were just not able to share each other's problems at that time.
But, to answer your question, what can one do? I think one simply has to be prepared to throw off the expectations of com-

panionship and dig in and become a caregiver. I think that's what one has to be prepared to do.

EZ: When I look back on it right now and ask myself, "How could it have been different for me?" I have no answer. I feel guilty when I'm sick, so of course I felt somehow that it was my own fault that I got the disease. I felt enormous pressure to shape up. I just felt very compelled to try to be OK. I had so many concerns which were over the top, like . . . this was aging me, I would never look the same, I would never be the same, I was old now, you would want someone younger, more attractive, you didn't want to be around any more illness. I think I was angry at you because I felt no real sympathy.

DS: The dilemma you were in was, you were my wife wanting to be treated like my wife, so you thought, but really wanting to be treated in a way I would treat my children or treat a casual friend. I do believe that I fell short, but you were angry at me all the time. It was hard to be there for you.

EZ: What's strange is that I only know *now* that I was angry at you *then*. I would have denied it at the time.

DS: But you were angry at everybody. You didn't like practically anybody during this period. You had negative things to say all the time about people. You just didn't seem to like people very much, which is not like you.

EZ: I don't remember that at all. I do remember feeling in a constant state of panic and fear. And yet also, at the same time, if you asked me how I was during that time, I thought I was all right. I think I presented as very strong. And there was a part of me that felt, *I can beat this; I can do this;* but I had to do it in some sort of isolation, I guess. I don't know that everyone on prednisone will feel as isolated as I did, and I don't really know what the anger was about. And I wonder if any of this was reflected in my performing, or my writing.

DS: I didn't see any difference in you as a performer. In general you seemed less vulnerable than you must have felt. You always seem very strong on stage, but I knew you were struggling. In terms of what you wrote during that time, I honestly don't recall. . . .

EZ: Well then, back to your advice for the companion of a person on prednisone?

DS: (pause, then . . .) If one's companion is on prednisone and develops a peculiar look in the eye, it's the prednisone. It's like a strange piece of personality that is ever on the alert for insult or harm. And another thing, I'd preface any emotionally loaded phrase with, "This may be the prednisone, but . . ."

The above interview with my husband, although brutally frank, made me appreciate how "different" I had become while I was on prednisone. David and I now are able to look back at that episode in our lives—when I was on prednisone and he was grappling with his own problems—as a really rough patch we have survived. In retrospect, it strengthened us, both individually and, now that we can talk about it openly, together.

In retrospect, I know that I was emotionally handicapped by the very medication that cured me. And yet I had to go on with my life and my work, muddling through as best I could. Although my best efforts to cope with rages and mood swings did not always meet with success, I was usually able to recognize when my response was "over-the-top." For example: When I experienced a flash of anger at something inconsequential, I could usually stop myself from blurting out some rageful remark I knew I would regret a second later. Often I was successful. Other times, regrettable words flew out of my mouth with little provocation. In an attempt to handle those outbursts, I began to develop some strategies. When I felt hot flashes of anger surge through my body, I actually told myself, "Cross the street." In other words, I tried to diffuse the situation instead of engaging in conflict. Sometimes I visualized myself walking

away to the other side of a road as I said the words to myself.
And sometimes it calmed me down, helped me think reasonably.

Dealing with sudden mood swings, with the highs and lows
of my emotions, was a constant challenge. When I was down,
I would try to remind myself that my misery was temporary, just
a momentary prednisone glitch. But knowing that a feeling had
been induced by medication did not make that feeling less real,
nor did it necessarily make it go away. Doctors' warnings about
the mood swings and emotional variables were essential, but
nothing really prepared me for the onslaught. While nothing de-
fended me completely, here are some suggestions from one who
coped as best she could with the exaggerated mood changes induced by this tough cure:

1) When you feel depressed, remind yourself that it's temporary. You are not sinking into a deep and bottomless pit of
misery. Actually say to yourself, "It's the medication. It's temporary."

2) When a rush of rage overwhelms you, defuse the conflict.
Let it go. Actually say to yourself, "Cross the street." Visualize
walking away. Don't engage in senseless tiffs.

3) Communicate with your loved ones and companions. Isolation does not help the healing process or nurture relationships.
Talk. And ask to be told when you're overreacting. In fact,
"you're over-the-top" might be a useful catchphrase for a family member to use, if it is used with affection.

4) Seek professional help. Do not, as I did, pretend to be fine
or try to tough it out alone. If you think you need help, you need
help. Get it. And remember that you will not need it forever.
This is temporary.

5) Do not hide behind the prednisone alibi, but when you
can't help it and you *do* blow your stack, try to learn from it so
you won't do it again. Apologize. Ask to be forgiven. "I'm
sorry; I'm not myself," is a good thing to say. And don't beat
yourself up. Forgive yourself. Then others will.

6) Do not sit home and examine how you feel every second. If you have spare time, read, write, watch videos. Reach out to friends. Spend time with other people, and don't talk about your illness. When you keep yourself busy and when you extend yourself to others, you keep the demons at bay.

7) Find ways to empty your mind. If you know how to meditate, you should do so often. If you have never meditated, you might try it.

8) Relax. There are books that offer helpful relaxation exercises, or you can create your own. I have several personal techniques that work well for me:

    a) I like to lie on the floor near a window, gazing up at the sky (or if I'm in a motel with a view of another building, I imagine the sky). Knees up, arms comfortably at my side, I think of space, openness, ease. I think of floating up into the sky. Sometimes I count to four, over and over; sometimes I repeat my personal mantra; and sometimes I visualize some beautiful outdoor spot.

    b) Lying on a bed or sofa, I imagine the mattress is a large meadow covered with soft moss and wildflowers. I imagine the feel of the warm sun on my face, the birds singing, a gentle breeze caressing me. I breathe deeply, and I am transported to a place that is calm and tranquil.

9) Whether or not you find relaxation techniques helpful, find time to "get horizontal." Lie down during the day, even if it's only for five or ten minutes. Allow yourself to let go of all worry. Forget about illness; forget your concerns. Let go of it all. Empty your mind of anxiety and fear. When you achieve moments of peace, you help yourself toward recovery.

11

Weathering Withdrawal: You Can't Stop Cold Turkey

Slow tapering from high-dose steroids is important. Too rapid withdrawal can cause a shock to the system, since you may have suppressed adrenal function. In addition, too rapid tapering can result in a flare-up of some medical conditions. This chapter is to help you cope with tapering steroids.

Julie

Why "Cold Turkey" Cessation of Steroids Can Harm You

When your doctor prescribes steroids in high doses, the benefit to you should far outweigh the risks. If you have questions about this, you should have a long, heartfelt talk about your questions and concerns, because steroids are among the most potent hormone medications that can be administered. Handling not only the side effects but the effects of weaning you from the steroids must be part of the treatment plan. You can't just stop steroids abruptly and expect to have everything go well. Here is why:

Taking steroids interrupts your body's normal "feedback" system between the pituitary gland, a little structure that sits at the base of your brain, and your adrenal glands, where steroids are made. Under normal, healthy circumstances, when your body needs to make more steroids for regular activities (physiological amounts), one of the signals to make more steroids comes from your pituitary gland. The pituitary produces and releases ACTH (which stands for adrenocorticotrophic hormone, a name that means "the hormone that tells the adrenal cortex to make steroids, including glucocorticoids"). The ACTH stimulates the cortex (outer portion) of the adrenal gland to make more steroids. Then, when enough steroids have been made for normal physiological activities, the pituitary turns off. This is called a feedback loop. The amount of ACTH circulating in your body is very small, and so are the amounts of steroids. These are called physiological amounts—just the right amount needed when everything is in balance.

Your own adrenals produce only tiny amounts of steroids compared to the amount generally supplied when you take pharmacological amounts of the stuff, as occurs when your doctor prescribes steroids. Prescribed steroids suppress or turn off the feedback interaction between your pituitary and your adrenals. If you were to stop the steroids suddenly, your adrenals would just dumbly sit there and not make enough steroids to keep your body in balance. This act would lead to acute lack of steroids, with resultant low energy, low blood pressure, increases in blood potassium, and shakiness that can culminate in a crisis situation with severe hypotension (very low blood pressure), cardiac arrhythmias (irregular heartbeats, from the high potassium), and even shock. This can occasionally even be fatal. Thus stopping steroids "cold turkey" can turn you into a cold bird indeed. For this reason, steroids need to be tapered, that is, the dose reduced as you are slowly "weaned off" the medicine. The specifics of tapering steroids should be discussed with your doctor. Even when the steroids are tapered properly, however, you may experience unpleasant "withdrawal symptoms."

Withdrawal Symptoms

The degree to which any one person will be troubled during steroid taper varies considerably. Some people notice very little, if any, change in anything. While this fortunate situation may be yours, Eugenia's feelings of fatigue, mood warps, bone pain, temperature intolerance, and a sense of loss of control are typical for many adults. Family and teachers need to know that a young child may not be able to explain how he or she feels. Instead the child may suddenly develop odd complaints and new behavior at home and at school. For example, a quiet child may become obstreperous or alternate between acting withdrawn and acting loud. The effects of withdrawal may occur every other day in patients who are on an every-other-day schedule. Here is a list of possible manifestations of steroid "withdrawal" effects. Note that the findings and feelings during steroid withdrawal are particular for each individual. You or a family member may not find any withdrawal symptoms or may find a set unique to you not listed here:

- Muscles, bones, joints: Soreness, aches, especially of the legs, often at night.
- Energy level: You may feel full of energy one day and completely exhausted the next.

- Appetite: Change in appetite: more (or less) on the day following the steroid dose; cravings for particular foods; aversions to particular foods. You may simply notice a gradual lessening of appetite.
- Gastrointestinal: You may have changes in how your "gut" feels, with "stomach aches" on alternate days. There can be some change in bowel habits. Any big change should be reported to your doctor.
- Mood: While patients are on high-dose steroids, moods can go up and down, and psychiatric symptoms can be florid in a few patients. During steroid withdrawal it is quite common to have mood swings, even if you didn't notice these before. You may simply feel "low" on the days in which steroid dose is absent. On the other hand, you may have big changes, hour to hour, in how you feel.
- Skin, sweat glands, hair: You may notice variations in the amount of perspiration you have, changes in hair growth or luster. You may start to see an improvement in problems you have had related to high-dose steroids.
- Eyes: Some people may find that they see better one day compared to the next.
- Menstrual cycle: If your periods were irregular or stopped on high-dose steroids, they may gradually become more regular as the dose decreases. Or they may become irregular now.
- Blood pressure: Blood pressure often decreases. If you developed high blood pressure on high-dose steroids, this may improve. In fact, if you have been requiring blood-pressure-lowering medicine, your pressure could even become too low.

It is important that you know about these various signs and symptoms. Ask your doctor to monitor you for these difficulties. Know that these things are usually transient and worth enduring to get on lower steroid doses or to "get off" steroids.

What If There's a Flare-Up of Your Illness While You Are on a Tapering Steroid Dose?

Depending on the reason that you are taking steroids in the first place, your doctor may need to increase your medication dose, perhaps substantially. If the flare-up of your illness is serious, it will no doubt be worthwhile to increase the medication dose. It is important that you talk to your doctor about the change in both your medication and your underlying condition. Since the range of illnesses for which glucocorticoids are prescribed is so large, it is impossible to suggest specifics here, but rather, I suggest that you satisfy yourself about the reasons for increasing the steroids.

If you had been tapered down to a low steroid dose and now have to be on high-dose steroids again, you should follow the same lifestyle changes that you found helpful when you were on the higher steroid doses before. Give yourself permission to feel upset about it, but then put one foot in front of the other and take care of yourself.

For some patients, tapering steroids is the hardest part of treatment. It seemed to be for my sister.

Eugenia   Under the care of Dr. Daniel Libby, I began lowering my dosage of prednisone slowly but steadily. Instead of weekly visits to his office, I now saw him every other week. My dosage was reduced by five milligrams every two weeks, so by the time I was into my fourth month on prednisone, I was taking thirty-five milligrams every other day. Having begun titrating down from sixty milligrams a day, my dosage was now reduced by about three-quarters. It was at this point that I began to experience some of the problems of withdrawal. First and foremost, I was very tired. When I asked my doctor about it, I was told that fatigue is normal during withdrawal. But this felt *abnormal*. The fatigue was overwhelming, knocking me down when I least expected it. This was such a flip-flop—for the first three months on high doses of prednisone I had been wired all the time, energetic to the point of sleeplessness. Now I was so exhausted, it was all I could do to walk to the corner. In an attempt to go with the flow instead of against it, I began to take short naps during the day, which helped me to slog through the exhaustion and to do my work. But there was another new problem: I noticed that my emotional highs and lows were more exaggerated. They were no longer mood swings. They were mood *warps*. I was hypersensitive, weepy or giddy, depressed or manic. I felt emotionally out of control. And then, into the fifth month on prednisone, when the dosage was down to thirty milligrams every other day, I began to experience yet another side effect of withdrawal: bone pain. My feet were killing me. I had constant aches and pains up and down my legs.

I questioned my doctor. "Some of my patients can hardly walk during withdrawal," Dr. Libby told me.

My bone pain was pronounced, but I walked. I even used the treadmill each day. I felt stiff and achy all over, but because I was eager to get off the prednisone as fast as I could, I pushed through the pain and the exhaustion and the mood warps without complaining too much. I also began to see a pattern: Each time I reduced the dosage by five milligrams, I would experience five rough days of crushing fatigue and exaggerated pains and mood swings, and then it would level off. My body would get used to the lower dosage, and I would begin to do better . . . until the next reduction. But recognizing that there would be a bad patch each time I lowered the dosage of prednisone helped me prepare to deal with the onslaughts. I even felt optimistic that my withdrawal was going so smoothly. I was out of the woods, or so I thought.

Then it was August, the dog days of summer, and I was down to twenty milligrams, when I suddenly began to cough. It was nothing, I decided, a mere little cold. But within a few hours, I was pulling for air, feeling my chest tighten. And I quickly called the doctor.

"I don't think this is a relapse," Dr. Libby said. "It's bronchitis." But because I had to travel up to Maine to play at a chamber music festival, he gave me antibiotics and said that I should temporarily increase my dosage of prednisone: fifty milligrams the first day, forty on the second, thirty the next, then twenty-five and back to twenty. I did as I was told, and, having suddenly upped the dosage, I felt stoned on prednisone again, able to breathe but wired to the max, and in a state of panic. I decided it was not bronchitis. It was my disease coming back. I had relapsed. I would be on prednisone forever. I felt defeated, like a failure. Doomed.

"You're over-the-top," I told myself as I drove my rented car from the airport in Portland, Maine, up the Intercoastal highway where, three hours later, I found myself in a tiny, airless room in a hotel, staring at a wall, feeling terrified. Somehow I got through my first rehearsal with my colleagues. I then drove to a grocery store and stood in the produce section for a very long time trying to remember what I had come to buy. Finally, I purchased fruits and yogurts and rice cakes, and, back at the hotel, I ate what I could, then lay on the bed, sweating in the heat, sleepless. By morning, I was a total wreck. My husband, David, arrived to save the day. He found me weeping when he entered the room. I looked up at him and asked, "Why am I here?"

I had never felt helpless before; but in Maine, back on high doses of prednisone, I was a pathetic mess. Lucky for me, David took charge. He helped me pack and moved me to much nicer, cooler lodgings. He held my hand and told me it was a temporary setback, that I would be fine. I felt better. Although my husband could only stay for one day, his presence calmed me down. I was able to enjoy the rest of my time in that beautiful seaside setting, even though I was jangled by sudden rushes of fear and trembling. The concerts were a challenge because on stage I experienced arbitrary moments of panic. But I kept telling myself it was the medication, not me; and I did the best I could.

When I returned home, I was able to reduce the prednisone quickly back down to twenty milligrams every other day, but it took me some time to feel better. My body seemed to be reeling, and I was worried. I feared getting sick again and having to go back yet again on megadoses of prednisone. Dealing with the fatigue, bone pain, and mood swings of withdrawal was bad enough. Now I felt the specter of relapse haunting my life. I never communicated my fears to my doctor. I wanted him to think I was doing well, coping with it all. Had I let him know how very high my level of anxiety was, he undoubtedly would have suggested I see a therapist.

Although I did not see a psychiatrist, I was helped during my withdrawal by a serendipitous conversation with a friend, a fellow musician, who had to take massive doses of prednisone for pericarditus (inflammation of the tissue surrounding the heart) for six months. She assured me that exaggerated responses were not uncommon during the withdrawal phase. In her case, she said, "if anyone said anything that contradicted my point of view, I would feel the most extreme internal fury. Or if people were not meeting my expectations, I would experience rage." She spoke of severe panic attacks, including one in particular—on a plane to Paris when there was mild turbulence and she experienced "profound terror," as if "someone were standing beside me with a machine gun."

Because of her panic attacks, my friend went to a therapist who helped her understand what was happening to her. He explained that during withdrawal from prednisone any stimulus to the adrenals sends them into a tizzy, and they produce either too little or too much adrenaline. He said that her panic attacks were not unusual and shared a story with her about a patient, a normally mild man, who was being weaned from prednisone. He apparently went to a grocery store and because the checkout line was too long burst into a mad rage, ripping items off the shelves, and had to be subdued.

I did not act out in a grocery store, but I think I might have, if provoked. Knowing that I was not alone in my off-kilter responses helped me avoid unraveling completely.

During this difficult period of withdrawal, I also experienced occasional dizziness and general weakness. I began to wonder whether I was becoming hypoglycemic, but before bothering my doctor with it, I found that drinking a glass of fruit juice when I felt shaky solved the problem. My diet was already high in protein, but I craved even more. Eating lots of chicken and fish seemed to make me feel stronger.

My legs and feet really hurt, and I was helped by a chance encounter with a massage therapist. I was performing at the Hollywood Bowl, in Los Angeles, and my back was killing me. The hotel offered massage service, so I indulged, and the strong Russian woman who came to see me suggested an exercise that would relieve pain in the lower extremities. She told me to lie on my back and bicycle in the air. I followed her directions, using a small pillow to elevate my buttocks so I would not strain my lower back. One hundred full cycles in the air, daily, seemed to help. Perhaps the nonresistance of this effort stimulated circulation. In any event, air-biking did bring me some relief . . . and probably tightened my stomach muscles as a bonus.

Instead of getting easier, withdrawal seemed more difficult the lower the dosage became. After ten milligrams, the reduction was in decrements of two and one-half milligrams. I stayed for three weeks at seven-and-one-half milligrams, then three weeks on five, and finally down to two-and-one-half milligrams. That small an amount of prednisone is negligible, but I stayed on it for six weeks and still felt its effects. The day I took my last little dose of prednisone, I celebrated, thinking, *Now I'll instantly be back to my old energetic self!* But it took another two months before I felt I had even begun to regain my vigor and my emotional balance.

All in all, I was "on prednisone" for ten months and felt its effects for another two. I only know now, after the fact, how truly tough my year of coping with this medication was; and the most challenging part of it all was during withdrawal.

12

The Future:
Life after
Steroid Treatment

Eugenia Six weeks after I stopped taking prednisone I played a concert in New Haven, and I was aware, on stage, that I finally felt good up there with my flute. I was not plagued during the performance by those sudden stabs of terror, mistimings, or odd visual glitches. I was prednisone-free and back to my old self again. Now all I had to deal with was my normal level of anxiety and neurosis. After the concert, I breathed a true and deep sigh of relief.

Until that concert, I had no real conception of how difficult it had been to perform while I was taking prednisone. It was as if an enormous weight had been lifted, and I felt airborne, euphoric. But I soon discovered that I was not entirely free from worries or potential problems.

Two months after I was completely finished taking prednisone, I received a phone call about changing the venue for a rehearsal for a chamber music concert. One of the player's daughters was sick with a cold and fever, and no baby-sitter was available. I was asked if I minded rehearsing in the sick child's home. I flashed back to my relapse in Maine, and I was instantly afraid that I would catch the cold, which would turn into bronchitis, and I would not be able to breathe and I'd have to go back to taking prednisone. "Hold it," I then told myself. "You're healthy now. Just don't kiss the kid, and you'll be fine. Take your vitamins. Go to rehearsal." I did. But my knee-jerk reaction underlined a fear that lingers and is hard to shed.

It also seemed to take a long time for my energy to return to normal, and I experienced occasional inexplicable mood twists for months after I stopped taking the medication. In order to feel truly well, I realized, it was important to stay strong and positive. To me, that meant taking care of myself, eating sensibly, exercising moderately. No longer on a restricted diet, I nonetheless decided to keep away from fats and sweets.

After I had been free from prednisone for four months, I had a bone density test, which revealed that I did not have any bone loss. I was delighted. As for lasting side effects, I still experience some pain in my feet, and I can still detect a change in my shape around the kidney area. I am told that both of these side effects should fade with time.

Dr. Libby tells me that I will not relapse, that my eosinophilic pneumonitis is history. But I've read the articles on it. It *does* recur. It *can* become chronic. I truly appreciate my doctor's optimism, and I want to believe him, yet I can't seem to delete a small file labeled "what if?" from the hard drive in my head. What if I relapse and what if I have to spend another ten months taking prednisone? The idea overwhelms me, but it does not terrify me. I have learned a great deal about the side effects of prednisone, and if my disease should (God forbid) recur, I will be armed to protect myself from its side effects. And I can always refer to this book.

13

Lessons Learned from a Tough Cure

Eugenia   It's early spring. Delicate green leaves unfurl on the trees in the park near my home. The daffodils and crocuses are up. The forsythia unfolds, and the cherry blossoms are about to burst open. Exuberance is in the air. Everyone is outside, and everything is in motion. Toddlers take their first steps; bike riders whiz by. Rollerbladers, skateboarders, walkers, and runners all whirl in the revelry of renewal, and I, alive and well, whirl too.

The earth's rebirth seems even more miraculous to me this year. Last spring I was seriously ill, gasping for breath, and although I am grateful for the medicine that made me well again, I'm nonetheless struck by the inescapable paradox of prednisone—that it is both a cure and a curse. The cure out-weighs the curse, but it is certainly one tough remedy. I cannot say I coped with it well. I merely did what I could to get through the rough parts. Having an advocate in my sister was invaluable, and our experience together has been both bonding and illuminating. Although we sisters live very different lives in different cities, our closeness has nonetheless always been a given. We've cheered each other's triumphs, soothed each other's sorrows, but my brush with mortality and Julie's instant and unfailing involvement in my recovery have given me a deeper understanding of our bond. It goes beyond sibling success and failure. It is both visceral and primal; it is, very literally, a bond *for* life.

I have been free from prednisone for two months now, and I often am amazed at the difference in how it feels to be "off the stuff." Now I can perform onstage or stand in front of the camera without fearing a sudden jab of nerves or a rush of terror. I no longer have wildly exaggerated responses to minor annoyances. My patience has returned and so have my energy, my optimism, my hopes and dreams. I wake up happy, thankful to feel good and to have the great fortune of another day on this earth. "As long as you have your health"—I used to roll my eyes when my elders said that. Now I nod knowingly.

When I look back, I am astounded that it took so long for my disease to be recognized. But I now realize that I was culpable for not acknowledging how truly lousy I felt. I blamed it all on having turned fifty, an assumption I now find not only diminishing but just plain stupid. Attention must be paid to symptoms, no matter what age you are. If your doctor does not see or hear anything and you have a gut feeling that indeed there really is something wrong with you, demand more tests, or consult a second doctor. Just because a disease cannot be seen or heard does not mean that there isn't something lurking like a stealth bomber in your body. At any time in our lives we have the right to expect our problems to be treated with respect. It is not acceptable when a doctor says, "What can you expect for a person of your age?"

My own father's battle with cancer should have taught me a lesson in demanding a diagnosis. He struggled valiantly with prostate cancer and refused to accept his death sentence without a courageous fight. Because he was an inventor, he used his scientific acumen to seek out and to demand cutting-edge treatments, and in so doing, he managed to extend his own life for five years longer than expected. He died like a warrior. Losing him taught me how evanescent life is, how very brief, and in his absence the lessons he taught me loom larger. He encouraged me to pursue all of my interests, and when I would ask, "But how will I get it all done?" his answer was, "Simply apply your ass to the chair." Do the work. That was his message. Battling a serious illness and surviving in good health has filled me with a sense of urgency to do the work, to get it all done, to do it well, to grow, to learn. I feel more privileged than ever to be able to apply my ass to the chair.

Because my disease threatened my ability to play the flute, I find that I now play it with more passion, more commitment. I approach my daily practice with renewed enthusiasm. I am filled with the joy of being able to express myself through this lyrical, incantatory instrument. When I remember how it felt to perform on prednisone I can only describe it in metaphors: it was like dancing on the third rail; it was like balancing on a wire over Niagara Falls; it was like walking through a jungle in the dark; it was like being alone at night in the bedroom of a house when you think you hear someone on the stairs. Now that I am free from prednisone, the stage is once again a safe haven. Rehearsals are like parties, and every concert feels like a celebration to me. I used to say that I wanted to play the flute until my teeth fell out. Now I want to play the flute until my lungs collapse. Maybe longer.

Besides a sense of urgency and commitment and renewed enjoyment in my work, I believe that there are some real lessons to be learned from a tough cure. First and foremost, I've learned that communication is key. I should have taken my symptoms more seriously. And then, once diagnosed with a serious illness and feeling that I had failed by "allowing myself" to get sick, I worked very hard at seeming to be well. I did not communicate my fears and concerns. I kept telling myself from the start that this illness was no big deal. In fact, my husband was out of town when I went to the hospital. I was by myself as I weathered the endless hours of CAT scans, x-rays, breathing tests, and blood work that led to a diagnosis.

"Why didn't you call me?" one friend asked when I said I had been alone at the hospital.

"Why? What's the big deal?" I asked back.

"The big deal," she answered, as if talking to a slow student, "is that it must have been frightening. Don't tell me you weren't scared."

"To death," I wanted to say, but I shrugged it off instead with, "Not really." I simply could not admit to myself that being very ill was terrifying, and therefore I did not express my true feelings or needs to those near me. I fault myself for not having told my first lung doctor when I felt particularly ill or weak. From the day of my diagnosis, I should have been more honest with him and with myself and with everyone around me. Instead, I instantly became very isolated. The upside of this downside was that I was forced to figure things out on my own. I stopped being a passive patient. I took charge of learning about my disease, about the medication and its side effects. Julie provided me with information, and together we forged a strategy for coping with probable side effects. We fashioned a diet; we figured out how I could exercise, how often and how much; we discussed how I was feeling, because she was my big sister the doctor and the one person to whom I could really talk about this illness. But I never told her how frightened I was.

When I changed doctors and became a patient of Dr. Daniel

Libby, I was able to talk more freely with him. He was open to questions; his gentleness and compassion helped me to be more honest, and soon my care began to seem somehow collaborative. I felt as if I was taking an active part in my own healing. I believe that as health care becomes less readily available to all of us, involvement in our own cure is crucial. If the lines of communication and cooperation remain open, the patient-doctor relationship strengthens. The job gets done with greater efficiency. When we as patients become more informed and more involved in our own care, it can only help speed recovery.

I recently went to Golden, Colorado, to perform with the Jefferson Symphony, and in that quaint mining town I met a woman who asked me what I was writing. I told her that I was collaborating with my sister the doctor on a handbook for coping with prednisone. The woman's eyes widened. "Why couldn't you have written it six years ago?" she asked plaintively. "I've been struggling with megadoses since then." We shared prednisone stories. Compared to her six-year-and-still-ongoing saga involving such side effects as severe eye damage (cataracts) and weight gain and clinical psychosis (for which she was taking medication), my voyage on prednisone was blessedly brief, and I had disembarked almost unscathed. But no matter how lucky I feel after the fact, during treatment I experienced the roughest ride of my life.

During my stay in Golden, I took an early-morning hike up Lookout Mountain with the conductor of the orchestra, Antonia Joy Wilson, a talented and very fit young woman. I, of course, led the way, and after a particularly difficult ascent up a switchback trail, I felt really winded. I was pulling for air; my chest ached. I was alarmed. Was my disease returning? Would I have to go back on prednisone? I was close to panic when Antonia yelled to me, "Could we stop for a minute, please? I can't breathe!" I turned to find her huffing and puffing just as hard as I was. I suppose I will always be on alert for signs of a relapse. I pretend that I do not fear it, but of course I do. And yet now I know that if I ever need to take megadoses of prednisone again, I'll be armed with this handbook to help me get through it.

It is my hope that this guide will offer comfort and constructive suggestions for other patients whose conditions must be treated with this miraculous yet monstrous medicine. I am aware that for a myriad of reasons there are some people for whom no prophylactic actions will help to avoid the side effects of prednisone. This handbook is, therefore, not meant to be a panacea, nor do I offer my participation as anything more than personal experience. But because shared experiences can lead to a collective wisdom, I have wanted to contribute my story of struggle and recovery.

Julie We physicians are taught to analyze, to speak in measured phrases in response to making a grave diagnosis. This response gets transformed to a kind of "bedside manner" approach to life, by which I can appear to respond with completely rational demeanor to almost anything, including frightening, dispiriting, or disconcerting news. This permits a certain remove that facilitates action. Yet it can get in the way of honest, from-the-gut reaction. There is likely an upside and a downside to this set of responses.

The upside with respect to Eugenia was that rather than becoming frantic with worry, I launched into action mode. I didn't know much about eosinophilic pneumonitis, but I found out what I could in a hurry. My job as a doctor means I am primed to make easy connections to other doctors, to find the most up-to-the-minute literature, and to get specialized help. So I could check up about what should be done, whether it was, in fact, being done, and whether Eugenia's doctors should do more. I could read up on treatments. I could talk to her doctors. I could help as a medical liaison. In the best sense, having a doctor for a relative may help the patient, as well as the patient's health-care team, in communication.

But there are *many* downsides. A doctor relative can be an interference, can subtly demand either too many studies or too few. A doctor in the patient's family can lead to overreaction or underreaction on the part of the treating doctor. Indeed, doctors' spouses often get the worst care because both the physician spouse and the treating doctor combine to treat the patient differently from the usual standard of care. In the worst instances, doctors demand too many opinions for and about their loved ones and end up with idiosyncratic or odd therapy.

As Eugenia's sister, I obsessed about what I was doing to help her with her disease after I blurted out, "I think you need more tests!" I began demanding that she be seen (or that her records and films be seen) by additional doctors in Boston, where I live and work. I had already spoken to colleagues who thought, even without seeing her x-rays or CAT scans, that she needed a lung biopsy. It turned out that she never had the biopsy or what we call a "full" work-up, and I still think she should have. Perhaps I should have insisted. Nonetheless, I feel confident that my consultation was useful.

I have learned a lot from my sister's illness. It has made me rethink my reaction to other family members' illnesses. I am an action person, and I always try to get involved when health-related problems occur in the family. I think I have been effective in some instances and worse than counterproductive in others. The unfolding of each instance has depended on the seriousness of the problem together with the approaches and personality of the particular family member, the treating physician, and my situation at the time. This set of circumstances is likely true for any doctor who finds him- or herself in this situation.

My mind returns to when my father first had prostate cancer and wanted to avoid surgery. He knew his cancer was an aggressive one (according to so-called Gleason staging), but he opted for irradiation. I did not "push" him into surgery, feeling that the outcome was likely to be bad no matter what. But I now wonder whether I should have, often thinking, *Yes, I should have.* I also did not talk at length to his doctors. This might have helped him in making a better decision.

With Eugenia, I wanted to be more involved. When I suggested she should have a biopsy, she balked and said, "Just because you couldn't save Dad, don't overdo it with me." Her comment infuriated me, but there was some truth to it. Yet, in her case, I felt I had more to offer because I often prescribe steroids and have dealt with their side effects.

There are some general lessons in our story, as well as the personal ones. The general lessons are that I, like any doctor, need to allow myself perspective with respect to family. As a doctor, I want to be sure that my loved ones have the care they need, and that once they have it, I can return to being a sister, a daughter, a mother. The relative-doctor needs to let the patient's doctor be the doctor. The relative-doctor needs to help (even push) the treating doctor to stay in charge. On the other hand, as a trained doctor, I shouldn't check my brains at the door. But neither should any patient or family member, even though not medically trained.

Eugenia's illness has led me to view the doctor-patient relationship differently. In the information age, the patient should be informed. The patient should be more than a passive recipient of treatment. I have come through this process to feel that the doctor-patient interaction, at its best, should be a collaboration for health.

The human thing I have learned is how much I love my sister. Our long-standing association, first due only to the random act of birth, has been strengthened over the years and now through Eugenia's illness and its necessary treatment. I have a big stake in helping her cope with it. In that sense, her illness's gift to me was to help me know that I am, in a sense, my sister's keeper.

14

Recipes
to Help You
Beat the Bloat

Eugenia NOTE: *Being on prednisone means being re-stricted to a limited choice of ingredients. The challenge is to be creative within those restrictions. The recipes offered here are ones that I challenged myself to concoct during my treat-ment with prednisone. I found that the key to cooking and en-joying food while on the medication was to vary the ingredients and buy the freshest foods available. When I tried to make each meal special, I did not feel deprived. Instead, I felt uniquely satisfied.*

I truly enjoyed each of the following recipes, but as we all know, taste is subjective. You will find your own way to creat-ing low-salt, low-sugar, low-fat meals that you love. I hope the recipes suggested here will inspire you and maybe even suit your taste too.

Basic Rules for Preparation

1) Do not add salt or sugar to any recipe. Also watch out for sodium chloride other sodium salts such as monosodium glutamate, sodium bicarbonate, et cetera, in food mixes and prepared food.

2) Use fresh herbs whenever possible. When using bottled spices, check the labels: prepared mixed spices often contain salt and/or sugar and other additives. However, there are excellent bottled salt-free herbs, made by such companies as McCormick and Mrs. Dash, with flavors like "Garlic and Herb" or "Lemon and Pepper" or "All-Purpose Table Seasoning." There are also salt-free mustards on the market.

3) Use olive oil for cooking and/or vegetable oil cooking sprays (my preference was olive oil cooking sprays).

Tips

1) Use a skillet with a nonstick surface. This helps minimize the amount of oil or cooking spray you'll need.

2) It helps to buy the following in quantity:
Lemons
No-sodium-added canned tomatoes and tomato sauce
Olive oil and nonfat cooking sprays

3) Buy a blender (or juicer) if possible.

4) Microwave. I found it to be the easiest way to cook things *fat-free*: vegetables, both frozen and fresh; fish; yams; fruits; et cetera. Also, by microwaving vegetables for 2–5 minutes, draining them, and then sautéing them, you use less oil and it takes less time.

NOTE: *Serving sizes are approximate. I always cooked more than I needed and stored the rest for another meal.*

Breakfast Treats

Your Basic Yam

As described in chapter 6, the yam is "among the most nutritious foods" available. I found that a hot yam with its warmth, sweetness, and smooth texture made a pleasantly filling and delicious breakfast meal.

INGREDIENTS:
1 large yam

To microwave: Wash the yam well. With a fork, pierce the yam in several places. Put it on a microwave-safe dish and cook on HI for 9–12 minutes, depending on size.

To bake in the oven: (The smell of a yam baking in the oven is lovely, and on a cold winter morning it will fill the kitchen with a sweet, fragrant warmth.) Preheat oven to 400°. Wash the yam well. With a fork, pierce the yam in several places. Put it on a cookie sheet (there will be some oozing, so tin foil placed on the cookie sheet can help minimize the clean up). Bake at 400° for 45 minutes. Slice the yam open. Sprinkle with coarse black pepper (for a tart flavor) or with cinnamon and/or allspice (for a sweeter flavor). Eat whole, skin and all, or scoop out the flesh with a spoon.

serves: 1

Hot Cereals

Eating a bowl of hot cereal can be very satisfying, even in warm weather.

INGREDIENTS:
Cereal (Wheatina, oatmeal, etc.)
Artificial sweetener
Fruits: berries or chopped fruits

Cook cereal as directed on the package, but use water instead of milk. *No* butter. *No* salt. Add artificial sweetener. Garnish with fresh berries or chopped apple, peach, or fruit of choice.

serves: 1

Yogurt with Warmed Fruits

The mixture of warm fruit with cold yogurt creates an agreeable sensation and brings out the flavor of each.

INGREDIENTS:
Fruit: 1 apple, peach, nectarine, or hard pear
1 8-oz container plain nonfat yogurt or "lite" yogurt (many
   brands of nonfat yogurt come flavored with artificial
   sweeteners, or you can do it yourself: add your own
   sweetener to plain yogurt, as well as a drop of flavoring
   such as vanilla, lemon, or almond extract)
Optional garnish: 1 T. unsweetened granola, sunflower seeds,
   or wheat germ

Slice the fruit. Place in a microwave-safe dish. Do *not* add water. Cover with a piece of paper towel or paper napkin. Microwave on HI for one minute (or more if the fruit has been in the refrigerator). Drain any liquid from the fruit. Spoon the yogurt over the fruit. Add a very small amount of garnish, if desired.

serves: 1

Yogurt Cheese

A simple do-it-yourself process that produces a tasty, tangy nonfat spreadable cheese.

INGREDIENTS:
1 large container plain nonfat yogurt (16-oz)

You can use a strainer, but for best results, use the filter cone from a drip coffeemaker. Line the filter cone (or strainer) with a paper cone filter. Spoon the yogurt into the paper filter. Place the filter cone (or strainer) over a container to catch the liquid from the yogurt as it seeps through. Cover the filter and place it in the refrigerator. Within 1 to 2 hours, the yogurt will be fully drained and congealed into "yogurt cheese." Discard the liquid, or drink it if you can. (It contains valuable nutrients but it tastes vile, to me.) Turn the yogurt cheese out into a bowl. You can add spices to it, such as pepper or a blend of salt-free spices and herbs. Spread on bread, rice cakes, crackers.

serves: 1–4

Breakfast Smoothie

A cool, satisfying drink, quickly made in the blender. It's filling, it's nutritious, and it's low in calories.

INGREDIENTS:
1 banana cut into large pieces (you can substitute other
*   fruits: mango, papaya, strawberries, peeled apple;*
*   experiment for preferred taste and texture)*
1 cup skim milk
2–3 ice cubes
Artificial sweetener
Optional garnish: cinnamon or nutmeg

Place all ingredients except garnish in the blender. Blend on HI until smooth (a few small chunks of ice may remain). Pour into a tall glass. Garnish.

serves: 1

Appetizers

Crudités with Yogurt Dip

If you like to nosh before dinner, this is a great nonfattening way to do it.

INGREDIENTS:

*Carrots, peppers (red, yellow, orange, green), cucumbers,
  broccoli, cauliflower, etc.)*
1 8-oz cup nonfat plain yogurt
½ cup chopped scallions
1 cup parsley leaves
1 lemon, freshly squeezed
Black pepper

Cut up the vegetables and arrange them on a platter. Put yogurt, scallions, and parsley in a food processor and process until the mixture is smooth and turns a bright green. Pour the mixture into a bowl and add lemon juice and pepper. Let sit for ½ hour. (If you want a dip with thicker texture, use yogurt cheese.)

serves: variable

Salt-Free Pickles

When I was a little girl, I loved pickles so much my Grandpa Morris nicknamed me Pickle Puss. Life without pickles is unthinkable, but while taking prednisone, I had to stay away from highly salted foods. And most pickles have tons. Julie sent me this salt-free pickles recipe which you might enjoy. (Because I was not using vinegar during my treatment, I remained pickle-deprived.)

INGREDIENTS:

3 to 4 fresh cucumbers
Several scallions
½ cup vinegar

½ cup water
2 T. oil
1 tsp. pepper-lemon mix
½ packet of artificial sweetener

Peel the cucumbers, and chop the scallions. Put into a quart container with ½ cup vinegar, ½ cup water. Add the oil. Add the pepper-lemon mix, and artificial sweetener. Let it sit for at least 2 hours before eating.

serves: 4

Salt-Free Popcorn

Delicious, satisfying, and low-calorie, popcorn is not only for TV watching. It is a fine pre-meal snack that is simple to make.

INGREDIENTS:
1 bag microwavable salt-free popcorn

Follow the instructions. Add pepper or a no-salt mixed spice or even drizzle with lemon juice.

NOTE: *You can prepare salt-free popcorn in advance and take it with you to the movies.*

serves: 1 or more, if you'll share . . .

Entrées for Lunch or Dinner

Breast of Chicken with Fennel, Ginger, and Garlic

This is a spicy dish; serve with plain, salt-free rice and a salad.

INGREDIENTS:
4 pieces boneless, skinless chicken breast
1 T. fresh ginger, grated
2 cloves garlic, crushed
½ lemon, freshly squeezed

Black pepper
½ cup fresh fennel, sliced in thin strips

Preheat oven to 375°. Place the chicken in a casserole dish. Mix the ginger with the garlic and add lemon juice. Spoon this mixture onto the chicken. Sprinkle with pepper. Top with fennel slices. Cover with tin foil. Cook at 375° for ½ hour. Remove tin foil and cook for another fifteen minutes.

serves: 2–3

Swordfish with Peppers and Onions

A colorful fish dish, easy to make, that goes well with a salad and a side dish of string beans or spinach.

INGREDIENTS:
1 lb. swordfish steak, cut into cubes
1 red pepper
1 yellow pepper
1 small onion
Juice of ½ lime
Coarse black pepper
Fresh parsley, chopped

Preheat oven to 375°. Place the swordfish in a casserole dish. Cut the peppers and onion into small pieces and place on top of swordfish. Top with lime juice and coarse black pepper. Cover with tinfoil and cook for 20 minutes. Uncover and cook for another 20 minutes, basting once or twice. Garnish with fresh parsley and serve.

serves: 2–3

Grilled Fillet of Salmon with Lime

A simple, delicious fish dish.

INGREDIENTS:
4 salmon fillets
½ lime

Nonfat cooking spray (if grilling)
Fresh black pepper
2 T. fresh dill, chopped

Preheat broiler. Prick the fillets in several places with a fork and pour the juice of ½ lime over them. Spray the grill with cooking spray. Place the fillets, skin side down, on the grill. Broil for 7–10 minutes, depending on the thickness. Remove from the grill. Add fresh pepper. Garnish with dill.

To microwave: Line a microwave-safe dish with paper towel. Place the salmon in the dish, skin side up. Cook on HI for 5–7 minutes. Turn upside down onto a plate, pour lime juice over fillets, add fresh pepper, and garnish with dill.

You can also grill (or microwave) swordfish steaks or other fish steaks using this recipe.

serves: 3–4

Grilled Lemon Chicken

An easy way to grill chicken and keep it moist and juicy.

INGREDIENTS:
4 pieces boneless, skinless chicken breast (flattened or not, as
*   preferred)*
¼ tsp. each of paprika and pepper
1 lemon, freshly squeezed

Preheat the broiler. Pierce the chicken with a fork in several places. Mix the paprika and pepper into the lemon juice and pour it over the chicken (you can do this earlier and marinate in the refrigerator). Grill for 5–7 minutes on each side, and during the grilling baste with more lemon juice.

serves: 3–4

Saucy Chicken Breast

*Chicken with tomato sauce, onions, and mushrooms. Delicious.
Serve with salt-free rice or pasta.*

INGREDIENTS:

*4 pieces of chicken breast (with skin and bones, or boned
    and skinned for lower fat content)*
Chopped onions
2 cloves garlic, chopped (optional)
¼ tsp. oregano
*1 medium can no-salt-added whole tomatoes or tomato
    sauce*
Sliced mushrooms
Nonfat cooking spray
1 lemon, freshly squeezed (optional)

Preheat oven to 375°. Place chicken breasts in a baking dish.
Mix chopped onions (and garlic if desired), dash of pepper, and
oregano with tomatoes or tomato sauce. Spoon tomato mixture
over the chicken and cover with tin foil. Bake at 375° for ½ hour.
Remove foil and continue to bake for 15 minutes.

Sauté sliced mushrooms in a skillet, using a small amount of
cooking spray. Top the chicken with the mushrooms when serving. Squeeze lemon over it, if desired.

serves: 3–4

Scallops and Nectarines

The citrus and shellfish combined creates a unique flavor.

INGREDIENTS:

1 lb. scallops
1 T. olive oil or nonfat cooking spray
1 clove garlic, peeled and minced
Black pepper
2 nectarines, sliced

1 *lemon, freshly squeezed*
Chopped fresh parsley

Wash and dry the scallops. Heat the olive oil or cooking spray in a skillet. Add the garlic and scallops and pepper. Cook over high heat, stirring, until scallops begin to brown. Add nectarines for the last few minutes of cooking time. Add lemon juice. Remove from heat and garnish with parsley.

serves: 3–4

Turkey Burgers

This dish goes well with grilled vegetables and a salad.

INGREDIENTS:
2 *egg whites*
⅓ *cup unsalted bread crumbs or rice-cake crumbs*
⅓ *cup fresh chopped onion*
2 *cloves garlic, minced*
1 *tsp. dried basil, crushed*
Pinch of dried tarragon
Pinch of dried mustard
Black pepper
1 *lb. skinned boned turkey or chicken breast, ground*
Nonfat cooking spray
½ *lemon*
Parsley sprigs
Lemon wedges (optional)

Preheat the broiler or start a fire in the barbecue grill. Beat the egg whites until they are foamy. Stir in the bread or rice-cake crumbs, onion, garlic, basil, tarragon, mustard, and pepper. Add the turkey or chicken. Mix well. Shape into ½-inch-thick patties. Spray the grill rack with cooking spray. Grill the burgers for 6–8 minutes or until done to your liking. Squeeze lemon on top, if desired. Garnish with parsley and lemon wedges.

serves: 3–4

Salmon Burgers

SEE: *Turkey Burgers. Simply substitute canned boneless low-sodium salmon for the turkey, but cook for only 2–3 minutes.*

Pasta with Olive Oil, Garlic, and Broccoli

INGREDIENTS:
1 *bunch broccoli*
1 *lb. pasta of choice (e.g., ziti, spaghetti, shells, penne, linguini, etc.)*
2 *T. olive oil*
2 *cloves garlic, chopped*
1 *tsp. dried rosemary*
1 *tsp. oregano*
⅓ *tsp. red pepper flakes (optional)*
4 *T. chopped Italian parsley (cilantro)*
1 *T. Parmesan or pecorino cheese*

Cut the broccoli into florets, peel the stems, and cut them into thin slices.

Read the package for cooking your choice of pasta. There are dried pastas that are sodium-free. You will want to watch the amount of pasta that you eat because of the sugars in carbohydrates.

Cook the pasta as directed on package and drain. As pasta is cooking, microwave broccoli for 3 minutes. Drain.

In a large skillet, heat 1 T. olive oil. Add garlic, rosemary, oregano, pepper flakes (if desired) and cook briefly. Add the broccoli, pasta, and cilantro. Add the other T. olive oil. Stir well. Put into a large bowl. Sprinkle cheese on top.

serves: 4

Pasta with Low-Sodium Tomato Sauce

You can create a variety of pasta sauces using the low-sodium tomato products available. Vary the vegetables you add and the kinds of pasta you cook.

INGREDIENTS:

1 *lb. pasta of choice*
1 *onion, chopped*
1 *yellow pepper, cut into pieces*
2 *cloves garlic, minced*
Olive oil or nonstick cooking spray
1 *large can no-sodium-added tomato sauce or whole tomatoes*
2 *scallions, chopped*
A pinch of red-hot pepper flakes, if desired
1 *T. Parmesan or pecorino cheese*

Cook the pasta as directed. While the pasta is cooking, brown the onion, yellow pepper, and garlic in olive oil or cooking spray for a few minutes. Add the tomato sauce or tomatoes, and stir until bubbling. (Add red-hot pepper flakes now, if desired.) Reduce heat and simmer until the pasta is cooked. Drain the pasta. Add the sauce. Top with chopped scallions. Sprinkle cheese on top, if desired.

serves: 3–4

Tofu and Vegetable Stir-Fry

Tofu is made from the protein of soybeans. It is a good high-protein substitute for chicken or fish, and combined with sautéed vegetables, it makes an excellent meal.

INGREDIENTS:

1 *lb. firm tofu*
2 *large tomatoes*
1 *onion*

1 *zucchini*
1 *large carrot*
½ *lb. sugar snap peas*
2 *T. olive oil or nonstick cooking spray*
½ *cup fresh basil, chopped*
Freshly grated ginger
Black pepper

Cut the tofu into large cubes. Cut up the vegetables, place together in a large microwave-safe bowl, and microwave them on HI for 3–5 minutes. Drain the vegetables. Heat 1 T. olive oil or cooking spray in a nonstick skillet. Sauté all the vegetables together, turning constantly, until they are browned. Add the basil, ginger, pepper, and the other T. of olive oil. Add the tofu, mix well, and cook, stirring occasionally, for another 3–5 minutes.

This dish goes well with no-sodium basmati or brown rice.

serves: 3–4

Salad Dressings and Salads

SALAD DRESSINGS

EZ's Basic Lemon Salad Dressing

Because I did not use vinegar (fermentation can cause yeast problems), lemon was a perfect substitute.

NOTE: *When you are eating out, ask the waiter for oil and some lemon wedges, and you can make yourself a tasty dressing. Top it off with fresh ground pepper.*

INGREDIENTS:
1 *cup olive oil*
½ *cup freshly squeezed lemon juice*
2 *cloves garlic, minced*

Pepper
Fresh dill
2 *T. fresh ginger, grated*
Fresh parsley
Chopped scallion

You can mix everything together in a bowl. However, my preference was first to coat the ingredients of the salad with olive oil (use a salad spoon at a time, and you will find that a little goes a long way). Add the lemon juice mixed with garlic and ginger. Toss the salad. Then add pepper, fresh dill, parsley and chopped scallion, and toss again.

serves: variable

Yogurt Salad Dressing

See "Yogurt Dip" above in "Appetizers." This dip also makes a great salad dressing.

Buttermilk Salad Dressing

This is a tangy dressing that goes well on all salads, but because buttermilk has added sodium use this dressing only once in a while.

INGREDIENTS:
½ *cup buttermilk*
2 *T. freshly squeezed lemon juice (or you can use cider vinegar)*
¼ *cup olive oil*
¼ *tsp. celery seed*
Black pepper
Dash of dried red pepper (optional)

Mix together and correct the seasonings to taste.

SALADS

Your Basic Mixed Salad

Here is a chance to test your creative mettle. Buy the freshest ingredients you can find. Wash everything well, and dry it well. Mix and match and toss yourself a tailor-made salad.

BASIC INGREDIENTS:
Lettuce—choose from the varieties offered
Carrots (use sparingly because of sugar content)
Cucumbers
Tomatoes
Endive
Arugala
Scallions
Broccoli florets
Cauliflower florets
Radishes
Celery
Sprouts
Watercress

ENHANCERS:
Tart apple, chopped
Water chestnuts, chopped (small amount)
Sunflower seeds, walnuts, almonds (small amount)
Garbanzo beans (small amount)
Sliced oranges or nectarines or grapefruit
Fresh uncooked peas

Sample Salad Idea: Watercress, Endive, Orange, and Walnut Salad

INGREDIENTS:
2 endives, washed and leaves separated
1 bunch watercress, washed well

EZ's Basic Lemon Salad Dressing
1　*orange, peeled and sliced*
1　*handful shelled walnut halves*

Put endives and watercress together in salad bowl. Toss with EZ's Basic Lemon Salad Dressing. Top with orange and walnuts.

serves: 3–4

SPECIAL SALADS

Chicken Salad with a Dash of Curry

This cold salad is lovely in the summer or any time. Flavored with a touch of curry, it is an exotic meal in itself.

INGREDIENTS:
1　*lb. boneless, skinless chicken breast*
1　*cup wild/long grain rice without salt*
Assorted cut vegetables: red pepper, onions, celery, carrots, fresh peas
Dressing (see below)
1　*handful sunflower seeds*

Poach the chicken in water for 10 minutes. Drain and chill.
　　Cook the rice. Drain and chill.
　　Add all the cut-up uncooked vegetables to the chilled chicken and rice.
　　Mix together and add dressing:
½　*cup olive oil*
Juice of ½ lemon (or vinegar, if allowed)
2　*cloves garlic, crushed*
Fresh ginger, diced
Black pepper
½　*tsp. curry powder*

Top with sunflower seeds and serve.

serves: 4

Shrimp, Snow Peas, and Roasted Pepper Salad

The warm peppers and snow peas give this salad a special zip.

INGREDIENTS:

1 *small head Bibb lettuce*
1 *lb. cooked shrimp, shelled*
2 *red bell peppers*
¾ *lb. snow peas*
1 *small red onion*
1 *tsp. no-salt mustard*
1 *T. freshly grated ginger (optional)*
1 *lemon, freshly squeezed*
Black pepper to taste
¼ *cup olive oil*
Fresh parsley, chopped

Wash and dry the lettuce. Wash and dry the shrimp. Preheat the broiler.

Cut up the red peppers and place on a nonstick cookie sheet. Place peppers under the broiler. Cook for a few minutes, turning the peppers until the skins are charred.

Microwave the snow peas for 2–3 minutes and drain. Chop the onion.

Place all of the above in a salad bowl.

In a small bowl, mix the mustard, ginger (if desired), lemon, black pepper, and olive oil. Stir in the parsley. Pour over the salad and toss. Chill and serve.

NOTE: *You can use low-sodium canned tuna or salmon in place of the fresh cooked shrimp.*

serves: 4

Vegetable Pasta Salad

Choose your pasta (any kind except spaghetti), cool it, and be creative with the ingredients. Again, because you need to watch your intake of carbohydrates, only enjoy a pasta salad occasionally.

INGREDIENTS:

Pasta of choice. Ziti or shells or penne work very well. Cook, drain, and chill for several hours, or overnight, if desired.

Mix and match any vegetables such as:

Red, yellow, orange, green peppers

Fresh uncooked peas

Uncooked broccoli florets

Uncooked cauliflower florets

Celery

Carrots

Onions

Scallions

Cherry tomatoes

Mix the chilled cooked pasta and raw vegetables. Toss with a low-sodium dressing.

NOTE: *You can add poached chicken pieces, cut-up leftover grilled salmon, or a can of low-sodium tuna or salmon to add protein to this salad.*

serves: variable

Vegetables and Side Dishes

Faux Fried Potato Slices

Once in a while, this neat trick with potatoes is a real treat, and it's low in calories.

INGREDIENTS:

Two large Idaho potatoes

Nonfat cooking spray

Black pepper to taste

Lemon wedges (optional)
No-sodium-added tomato paste (optional)

Preheat the oven to 400°. Wash and dry the potatoes. Cut into thin slices (¼ inch thick). Spray a cookie tray (or two, if needed) with nonfat cooking spray. Arrange the potato slices side by side on the tray(s). Place in the oven. Cook for 10–15 minutes or until the tops begin to brown. Carefully turn the potato slices over and cook until browned. Sprinkle with black pepper.

NOTE: *I liked to squeeze lemon onto these chips. If you have a yen for catsup, do not use regular tomato catsup, which has a high sugar and sodium content. You can use a no-sodium-added tomato paste instead.*

serves: variable

Roasted Vegetables

Roasting sliced vegetables in the oven at a high temperature will caramelize the natural sugars and make the vegetables taste extra-special.

INGREDIENTS:
1 small eggplant
1 zucchini
1 yellow pepper
1 small onion
1 fat carrot
Nonfat cooking spray

Preheat oven to 400°. Slice the vegetables in large pieces. Spray a cookie tin with cooking spray. Roast for 20 minutes, turning occasionally. Cook longer for crisper results.

NOTE: *Vary the vegetables according to availability.*

serves: 2–4

Spaghetti Squash with Tomato Sauce and Pignolia Nuts

The flesh of a cooked spaghetti squash can be pulled apart to form slender strands that resemble spaghetti. It is low in calories, has a crunchy texture, and makes a delicious side dish (or entrée, if you like). Topped with tomato sauce, it's delicious.

INGREDIENTS:

1 *spaghetti squash*
1 *8 oz. can no-sodium-added tomato sauce*
1 *handful pignolia nuts*
Black pepper

You can bake, boil, or microwave a spaghetti squash. Because the shell of the squash is so difficult to cut when uncooked, I find it easiest to combine microwave and baking as follows:

Preheat the oven to 350°.

Pierce the shell of the squash with a fork in several places.

Place on a microwave-safe platter and cook in the microwave on HI for five minutes. This will make it easier to cut the squash open. Remove the squash from the microwave oven and, using pot holders or other cloth to keep from burning yourself as you handle the squash, cut it in half.

Remove the seeds.

Place both halves of the squash, flesh side up, on a cookie sheet.

Bake in the oven for approximately 45 minutes to 1 hour, depending on the size of the squash.

While the squash is cooking, heat up the tomato sauce. You can also add vegetables to the tomato sauce, such as chopped onion, peppers, or zucchini.

Remove the squash from the oven. Let it cool or, using pot holders, take a fork and remove the flesh, which will easily separate into strands, into a large serving bowl.

Pour the tomato sauce on top of the spaghetti squash. Mix together.

Garnish with pignolia nuts and black pepper.

serves: 2–4, depending on size of squash

Beverages

Iced Herbal Tea

Make a double-strength pot of your favorite herbal tea. Suggestions: Mango, peach, peppermint. Pour over ice cubes and sweeten with artificial sweetener.

Herbal Tea Slush

Again, make a double-strength pot of your favorite herbal tea. Suggestions: cranberry, apple-orange, peach, peppermint. Empty a tray of ice cubes into a blender. Cool the tea prior to pouring a cup or so onto the ice. Then add 1 to 2 packets of artificial sweetener. Blend until frothy.

serves: 1 or 2

VEGETABLE JUICES/SHAKES

Health food stores make wonderful fresh vegetable juices, but not everyone lives near a health food store. If you have a juicer, you can make delicious fresh vegetable juices, without the added salts of prepared juices. Most juicers come with recipes and suggestions. I found fresh juices, like a mix of carrot, beet, and celery, to be truly satisfying snacks, full of vitamins and minerals.

There are many vegetable shakes you can make in a blender. For example:

Lemon Tomato Carrot Shake

INGREDIENTS:

1 *large carrot*
1 *cup plain nonfat yogurt*
⅔ *cup drained canned no-sodium-added tomatoes*
1 *tsp. lemon zest (yellow part of rind, grated)*
2 *ice cubes*

Trim and peel the carrot and cut it into medium-sized chunks. Microwave the carrot pieces on HI for 4–5 minutes. Drain.

Place cooked carrot in blender and puree. Add yogurt, tomatoes, lemon zest, and ice cubes into blender. Process on HI, scraping down the sides of the container with a rubber spatula, if necessary, until it's the consistency you like.

serves: 1

Squashed Squash Smoothie

INGREDIENTS:

½ *cup cooked, chilled butternut squash*
2 *T. soft tofu*
½ *cup skim milk*
pinch of cinnamon or allspice (optional)

Combine the squash and the tofu in the blender and process until smooth. Add the milk (and spice, if you like). Blend until creamy.

serves: 1

Cucumber Frappé

INGREDIENTS:

1 *cup plain nonfat yogurt*
½ *cup peeled, seeded cucumber, cut into chunks*
Mint sprigs
2 *ice cubes*

Combine all the ingredients in a blender and process until well blended.

FRUIT SMOOTHIES

Skim milk, or low-calorie juice, plus fruit, plus a few ice cubes can provide you with a terrific drink to enjoy at any time of the day.

SEE ALSO: "Breakfast Smoothie" on page 134.

Cranberry Rapture

You can use other low-calories juices besides cranberry to create a drink like this.

INGREDIENTS:
1 *cup low-calorie cranberry juice*
½ *cup skim milk*
2 *ice cubes*
Sprig of mint

Place all of the ingredients into the blender and process on HI until it's the consistency you like.

serves: 1

Peach Shake

You can also use nectarine for this recipe.

INGREDIENTS:
1 *large peach*
½ *cup plain nonfat yogurt*
¼ *tsp. vanilla extract*
Pinch of cinnamon
2 *ice cubes*
Artificial sweetener

Peel the peach; quarter and pit it. Put everything in the blender and process on HI until it's the consistency you like.

serves: 1

Kiwi-Banana-Strawberry Delight

The color of this shake is almost as much fun as its taste.

INGREDIENTS:
1 *kiwi*
½ *banana*
1 *cup sliced strawberries*

½ *cup skim milk*
2 *T. plain nonfat yogurt*
Artificial sweetener to taste
2 *ice cubes*

Peel the kiwi and banana; cut into chunks. Put everything into the blender. Process until it's the consistency you like.

serves: 1

Desserts

NOTE: *While on prednisone it is best to avoid dessert. But when the urge is overwhelming, try to stick to fresh fruits that have low natural sugar content.*

Mixed Fresh Berries

This is a colorful, low-calorie, low-sugar dessert that can be pleasing to the eye and the palate.

INGREDIENTS:
1 *cup blueberries*
1 *cup strawberries*
1 *cup raspberries*
Fresh mint

Wash, drain, and dry (place on paper towel) the berries. Remove the tops of the strawberries. Place in a pretty bowl and top with mint sprigs.

serves: 3–4

Broiled Grapefruit with Raspberries

INGREDIENTS:
1 *grapefruit*
½ *cup raspberries*

Artificial sweetener, if desired
Fresh mint

Cut the grapefruit in half. Section it. Place under a broiler for 3 minutes or in the microwave on HI for two minutes. Remove from heat, and garnish with raspberries. Sprinkle with sweetener. Garnish with mint.

serves: 1

Warmed Apple and Pear Slices

You can get the taste of a fruit pie without the crust just using sliced, fresh apples and pears. Warming them makes them taste sweeter. I found that the slices tasted great without sweetening, but you can add artificial sweetener to taste.

INGREDIENTS:
1 granny smith or other tart apple
and/or
1 fresh pear
¼ tsp. cinnamon
Artificial sweetener

Cut the apple and/or pear into thin slices, starting at one side and cutting inwards, so that rounds are formed. (This works better than cutting the fruit into quarters or eighths.) Place on a cookie sheet and heat at 300° for 10 minutes. Or, heat in a toaster oven until the fruit is soft. Sprinkle with cinnamon to taste. You may want to sprinkle artificial sweetener to taste. Or, microwave for 3 to 4 minutes on high.

serves: 1

Frozen Banana

This treat must be prepared in advance. It's a great way to make use of ripe bananas. But note that this dessert should only be eaten occasionally, because of its high natural sugar content.

INGREDIENT:
1 *ripe banana*

Peel the banana and place in tin foil. Wrap carefully. Freeze.

Roll the tin foil to the bottom of the banana and eat it like a popsicle.

serves: 1

STORE-BOUGHT TREATS

I did not have time to make my own sugar-free confections, so I made use of the marvels available at the grocery store, both ready-made and packaged.

Sugar-Free Gelatin

Look in the diet section of your grocery store for packets. To make, follow the directions. This is a fat-free, sugar-free treat that is also low in sodium.

Sugar-Free Candy

Many different kinds of sugar-free candy are found in your grocery store. Most are sweetened with sorbitol, which is non-absorbable, meaning that it will attract fluid into your intestines. Eat this candy sparingly. While it is delicious, eating more than 2 or 3 pieces is likely to cause increased frequency of bowel movements, or even diarrhea. (Because of this side-effect, sugar-free candy can treat constipation.)

Store-Bought Frozen Delights

Check your grocery frozen foods section for fat-free, sugar-free treats that you can indulge in when your sweet tooth overwhelms you.

For example:

Dannon makes a delicious nonfat frozen yogurt sweetened with Nutrasweet.

Weight Watchers makes some fat-free frozen confections that have a low sodium content.

15

Exercises

Eugenia When I was taking prednisone, I sometimes felt like a victim of the cure, instead of like a lucky patient who was taking a miracle drug. Controlling my diet was one way to feel less victimized. Exercising was another effective way to gain a measure of power. Not only did it give me a sense of regaining my strength, but it also made me feel that I was combating some of the potential side effects of prednisone.

Bone loss and the loss of muscle mass are two side effects of prednisone that you can help minimize by exercising. Depending on the nature of your illness or condition, you can find ways of moving and stretching that will help keep your bones and muscles toned and strong. Ask your doctor what, if any, your physical restrictions are and begin to craft a daily regime for yourself.

Since I am neither a physical therapist nor an exercise expert, I can only offer my own stretches and exercises as an example of one patient's attempt to counteract prednisone's physically depleting side effects.

EZ's Exercise Routine

From the age of eighteen, when I was first plagued with a chronic back problem, I began a habit of rolling out of bed in the morning, lying on the floor, and starting my day with stretches. I feel more supple and agile after stretching, ready to start my day. My back problem has not been solved, but it has been decidedly lessened, in large part, I believe, because of exercise and attitude. After seeing orthopedists who suggested spinal fusions and other invasive procedures, I consulted with a medical doctor who also had a background in chiropractic and acupuncture. His advice to me changed my attitude and helped me deal with this chronic problem. "You can see yourself as a fragile person with a structural problem that will only get worse," he said. "Or you can see yourself as a healthy person who can exercise and get stronger." Needless to say, I chose the second option and began to exercise with greater focus. My own stretch routine is therefore stress-free and strengthening for the lower back. It is also culled from an eclectic variety of sources— the orthopedist/chiropractor/acupuncturist, dance lessons, exercise classes, friends, even magazine articles. I divide the stretches in two parts: floor stretches and standing stretches.

NOTE: *The number of repetitions listed are simply a suggestion. Do as many or as few as you can.*

On the Floor

1) *Floor position one*

Lie on your back (on a rug or on a thin exercise mat), arms spread comfortably out at your sides, knees bent, feet on the floor, hip-width apart. Spend a moment aligning yourself. Lengthen your neck. Think of your spine elongating. Relax. Breathe deeply. Then follow these directions:

a. *Buttock squeeze.* Slowly squeeze buttocks together, hold tight for a few beats, then slowly release. Repeat ten times.

b. *Pelvic tilt.* Gently tilt pelvis forward and up until buttocks are raised a few inches from the floor. Slowly lower buttocks. Repeat ten times.

c. *Slow "bicycle."* Lie on your back. Put a pillow under your butt. Then slowly move your legs as if you are on a bicycle: Slide your right leg straight out down to the floor, keeping left knee bent. Inhale and bring the right knee toward your chest; exhale as you slowly straighten your leg up toward the ceiling. Do not lock your leg into a "straight" position; rather, keep it elongated, with your knee loose. Slowly lower your *elongated* right leg to the floor. Now do the same thing, starting with your left leg. Repeat ten times.

NOTE: *Remember to keep your pelvis and lower back pressed into the pillow. Move your leg in one continuous motion, resting as necessary at the start position (leg elongated).*

d. *Tracing a "circle."* Lower and straighten right leg. Bend the right leg, bring the knee up toward your chest, extend the leg straight up, then gently lower it comfortably out toward the right side of your body at an oblique angle, keeping your lower back and pelvis pressed to the floor; trace an arc back down toward the start position. Lower and straighten left leg, and proceed as above. Repeat two to five times.

e. *Leg and arm oppositional stretch.* Lower your right arm close beside your body. As you slowly stretch your right arm above your head, keeping it close to your ear, slide your left leg onto the floor and straighten it. Stretch your right arm up along the floor and left leg down along the floor, as if each limb is gently being pulled away from your body. Relax. Lower your left arm; slide your right leg to the floor. Repeat five times.

f. *Knee hug.* Bring your right knee to your chest. Wrap your arms around the knee. Inhale and raise your head up to your knee, hugging it toward your chest. Release knee and arms to position one. Repeat ten times. Do the same thing with left knee.

2) Floor position two

On your back cross your arms behind your head, elbows relaxed, knees bent, feet on the floor, hip-width apart. In this position, follow these directions:

a. *Modified sit-up.* Inhale deeply, then, as you exhale, pull in your stomach muscles and raise your cradled head and torso a few inches off the floor. Take another deep breath, and from this raised position slowly bring your torso up approximately five to ten inches more, hold a beat, then lower to the raised position. Take another deep breath and repeat. Repeat ten times. Lower your head on your crossed arms and rest.

b. *Oblique modified sit-up.* Cross your right leg over left. Lift your cradled head and arms to the raised position. Take another deep breath. Exhale as you reach your left elbow in the direction of your right knee. (Do not try to touch elbow to knee. This is a directional move.) Return to raised position. Now do this with your left leg. Repeat ten times.

c. *Ceiling reach.* From floor position two, lift your cradled head to the raised position. Take a deep breath. Turn your head and torso toward the right corner of the ceiling. Lift your torso up approximately five to ten inches toward that corner. Now repeat the same on the other side. Repeat ten times.

3) *Floor position three*

Take a small pillow and place it under your buttocks. Lie on your back, arms spread comfortably out at your sides. Keeping your feet relaxed, slowly "bicycle" your legs in the air. You will feel this in your thigh muscles, but you should feel no strain on your lower back. Do as many cycles as you can without straining yourself. Then, in order to stretch out your leg muscles, elongate your right leg, keeping the left bent, and in the air, and lower your right leg slowly to the floor. Feel the muscles relax, then raise the right leg back into a bent position. Now elongate your left leg, lower it to the floor, feel the muscles relax, and bring the left leg back into a bent position. Hug both knees to your chest. Release.

4) *Floor position four*

Lie flat on your stomach. Fold your arms and place your forehead comfortably on your folded arms. Follow these directions:
a. *Alternating leg raises.* Keeping your right leg straight but not locked (i.e., slightly bent if necessary), lift the leg up behind you a few inches and hold it there for a few beats; then lower it. Repeat with your left leg. Repeat this alternation ten times.
b. *Upper body strengthening raises.* Rotate your legs outward at the hip joints. This will give you better balance on your belly and pelvis, and there will be less stress on your lower back. Take a deep breath and, arching your back, raise your head (pillowed in your arms) a few inches off the floor. Hold and release. Repeat ten times.

5) *Floor position five*

On your knees sit back onto your heels and drop your head and arms forward onto the floor. Stretch your arms out in front of you, as if you are "praying toward Mecca." Follow these directions:

a. *Curled position stretch one.* Take a deep breath and as you exhale, slide your arms out on the floor away from your head, stretching gently. Inhale and relax into your curled position. Repeat five times.

b. *Curled position stretch two.* Take a deep breath and, pulling your stomach in, feel the back muscles lengthen and stretch.

c. *Cat curls.* From position five, push back with your hands and rise slowly, supported by your arms, until you are up on your hands and knees. Take a deep breath and round your back like a cat; exhale as you pull your stomach muscles in. Hold for a few seconds. Inhale and relax your back. Exhale and gently arch your back. Hold for a few seconds. Repeat five alternations.

d. *Jackknife leg stretches.* From your position in c on your hands and knees, curl your toes under and rock back and up onto your feet, pushing with your hands until you are in a "jackknife" position (hands and feet on floor, butt up in the air; do not lock your knees or elbows). Bend your right knee as you straighten your left. Feel the left hamstring stretch. Then reverse, bending your left knee and letting your right leg straighten. Repeat alternations slowly five times.

e. *Monkey swings.* From your jackknifed position in d, keep your knees slightly bent and walk your hands back toward you until you are balanced on both feet without hand support. You are still bent over, back rounded, head dangling, relaxed. Let your arms swing gently at your sides, monkeylike. Take a deep breath, place your hands on your knees for balance, and, keeping your pelvis tucked under, slowly uncurl to a standing position.

Standing Stretches

1) *Overhead reaches.* Stand with your feet hip-width apart, knees loose, arms relaxed. Spend a moment aligning your body. Inhale deeply. Exhale and let your shoulders relax; then let your

neck relax. Now bring your hands up to shoulder level and begin to alternately reach overhead. Do this easily, reaching straight up at first, then obliquely toward alternate corners of the room. Now make the movement larger: when you reach for the left corner of the room with your right arm, bend your left knee slightly and stretch up, rolling up onto the ball of your right foot. Now reverse. Enjoy the rocking motion of this stretch. Repeat as long as you like.

2) *Bending over.* Legs hip-width apart, begin by lowering your head. Keeping your pelvis tucked under, bend forward and downward, letting your arms dangle in front of you, keeping your knees slightly bent. Place your hands lightly onto the floor. (Bend your knees as much as you need to in order to touch your hands to the floor.) Gently shake your head as you would if you meant "yes." Now gently shake your head as if you meant "no." Place your hands on your knees for support as you gently roll up to standing, uncurling yourself upward like a fern. Repeat four times.

3) *Leg overhangs.* Legs hip-width apart, bend forward, but instead of between your legs bend forward over your right leg, keeping your knees straight but loose. Let your arms dangle until they touch the floor in front of your right leg. Inhale and feel the stretch in the right leg. Exhale. Inhale and exhale again. Now move your torso and arms over the left leg. Touch the floor in front of your left leg. Exhale. Inhale and feel the stretch in your left leg. Exhale. Inhale, and as you exhale again center your body, place your hands on your knees, and roll slowly up to standing. Repeat this sequence twice.

4) *Lunges.* Lean forward over your right leg as you have for the leg overhangs (3). Placing one hand on either side of your right foot, turn your feet and body forty-five degrees to the right. Now you are hanging over your body with the right foot in front of the left in a walking position. Supporting yourself with your hands on the floor on both sides of your right knee, allow your

left leg to slide out behind you until you are in a lunging position. Bend your right knee and loosely straighten your left leg behind you and feel the stretch. Keep your head aligned with your spine. Inhale deeply. Exhale. Bring your left leg back in, next to and parallel to your right. Turn your feet and body back to center. Now reverse the procedure: Place both hands on either side of the left foot. Turn your body forty-five degrees to the left and allow your right leg to slide out behind you in a lunging position. Proceed as you did for the lunge to the right. Bring your right leg in, next to and parallel to your left. Turn your body back to center and slowly roll up to standing. Repeat once.

Standing Upper Body Strengtheners

NOTE: *These arm exercises can be done with weights. When I was on prednisone I did not feel strong enough to use weights, but I found that doing these exercises carefully and with resistance, as if I had one-pound weights in each hand, seemed beneficial nonetheless.*

1) *Bent arm squeezes.* Bring both arms out to the side, elbows bent, arms up in a forty-five-degree angle (a "hands up" position) with arms held slightly below shoulder level. Squeeze both arms together in front of you (with resistance) until forearms and elbows meet, and open to starting position smoothly. Repeat twelve times.

2) *Back squeezes.* Bring both arms out to the side slightly below shoulder level, elbows bent, forearms in front of you, palms facing down. Squeeze your elbows (with resistance) down toward your waistline. Return to start position. Repeat twelve times.

3) *Upper back slides.* Bring both arms out to the side slightly below shoulder level, elbows bent, forearms in front of you parallel to the floor, palms facing down (as in 2). Reach both arms forward and slide them back, keeping them parallel to the floor,

until elbows are behind you. You will feel the deltoids contract. Slide arms forward as if along the top of a table until you are at the start position. Repeat twelve times.

4) *Rowing.* Bend both arms and bring your fists together at waist level as if you are about to row a boat. With a rowing motion, row your fists up to chest level, and feel your arms press up against your shoulders. Repeat the rowing motion twelve times.

5) *Triceps extensions.* Stand with knees slightly bent, feet hip-width apart, with your arms behind you, elbows bent. From the elbows, extend your arms behind you. Repeat the extension (or the opening and closing of the arm) as if it is hinged at the elbow. Repeat twelve times.

6) *Biceps curl.* Stand squarely, arms at your sides. Bend the arms up at the elbows, curling your fists (or weights) up to your shoulders. Slowly open and close the "curl" to work the bicep. You can alternate arms if desired. Repeat twelve times.

7) *Stretching out after doing these upper body exercises:*

    a. Cross your right arm across your chest and hug it close into your body with your left hand. Hold for a few moments as you inhale and exhale. Now cross your left arm across your chest and hug it in with your right hand close to your body. Breathe in and out slowly.

    b. To stretch the tricep, raise your right arm up over your head and let the forearm dangle down behind your head, elbow raised up in the air. Use your left hand to gently pull the elbow behind your head toward the left. Hold there. Breathe. Release your arms. Now raise your left arm up over your head and let the forearm dangle down behind your head, elbow raised up in the air. Use your right hand to gently pull the elbow behind your head toward the right. Hold there. Breathe. Release.

    c. Raise both arms above your head and clasp your hands. Stretch comfortably to each side a few times. Release your hands and bring your arms down to the side. Inhale deeply and exhale.

Swimming

For toning your body, swimming is a terrific exercise. If you have access to a pool, and if you have your doctor's approval, take advantage of the benefits of being in the water. Swimming is invigorating; and best of all, it does not put stress on your skeleton the way weight-bearing exercises do. You can do laps, try some water aerobics, or just "jog" at waist level across the shallow end of the pool. For me, nothing is quite as relaxing as the weightless wonder of floating on my back in water. Swimming reduces stress. You don't need to go to a beautiful beach or a spectacular lake to enjoy the benefits. Swimming anywhere is good medicine for the body and the spirit.

a) Hold a kick board and use a flutter kick for 2 to 4 lengths.

b) Do different strokes, being sure that you rest if tired.

Increase your work-out by one or two lengths/week.

Weight-Bearing Exercises

It is important when you are on prednisone to walk (or even run if you can) or bicycle, so that you strengthen the bones and muscles in the legs, hips, and pelvis. If you are well enough to do some low-impact aerobics, those would be beneficial. If you cannot get to a class, there are excellent videotapes available for you to use at home.

    I enjoyed walking and using a treadmill to walk during my prednisone therapy. Not only did it seem to kick-start my metabolism, but I really felt better after working up a sweat. Follow your doctor's advice for exercise. Don't overdo it. But if you are given a green light by your doctor, take a walk, a hike, a bike ride. Look at the flowers, enjoy your surroundings, and know that you are helping to heal yourself.

16

Partnership for Health: A Reexamination of the Doctor-Patient Relationship and Prescribing Practices

Julie Science and medicine have changed greatly during this century with the advent of antibiotics, the development of vaccines for many diseases, the cracking of the genetic code, and the invention of new technologies such as the laser. And with the discovery and synthesis of steroids. When the twentieth century started, doctors could offer little to patients compared to what present-day physicians can. Life expectancy has increased by more than ten years per person since then, and even genetic therapy is possible for a few diseases.

When I started medical school thirty-some years ago, learning the barest outlines about the genetic code seemed to place a physician on the cutting edge. Now, thanks to technology and the pervasive nature of TV, the use of DNA fingerprinting in the courtroom, the mapping of inherited diseases, and the possibility of gene therapy are known to most junior high school students. There are those who have a lot of negative things to say about the possible misuse of all of these advances. But there is a lot that is positive.

Along with the changes in medicine since the introduction of steroids have come the Internet and the World Wide Web. Both you, the patient, and I, the doctor, can access all sorts of experts to get advice about the most serious as well as the most trivial of problems. Indeed, in the computer age in which we live, you, as a patient, have access to all kinds of information about your health. And I, as a doctor, have the possibility of getting up-to-the-minute information about breakthroughs, problems, and new practices.

All of these advances have changed things for doctors. At the turn of the century, physicians offered support and did what they could. They made home visits and empathized; but without even antibiotics they often could not do very much to affect the course of serious infections or other serious maladies. Today hand-holding and home visits are rare, and technology has taken over. Doctors practice in groups, even in large "health maintenance organizations." The doctor you have today may not be on call or may not even be there tomorrow.

The practice of medicine has changed a lot, too, in keeping not only with advances but also, unfortunately, with the regressive realities of insurance limitations and ever-increasing bureaucracy. The bureaucracy of medical care can be overwhelming for patients, and for doctors, too. This bureaucracy is having an increasingly large effect on your health care. Even the concept of "health-care delivery" has changed. You, the patient, are a "consumer," while I, the physician, am a "provider." As a doctor I don't like to think of my patients as consumers and of myself as a provider—no matter what anyone says or writes. I prefer to think of myself in a partnership for health with patients. With limitations imposed all the time by creeping bureaucracy and pressure to see more patients in less time, it is important to set the stage for the best possible sharing of information.

There is much sophisticated information that you can obtain from multiple sources. The downside notwithstanding, you can and should be a well-informed patient. Here is what makes sense to me as a doctor:

- **You, the patient, should have as much information as possible about your condition.** Studies about how well patients follow through in taking care of their diagnosed health problems show that people remember best and comply with proper care if they get to talk about the particular issue with the doctor first and then get written information to take home. In other words, you hear the information directly and then you can review it again at home. This has clear implications for you.

  If you have to be on steroids, you should be sure you understand why the medicine is being prescribed. You should be an advocate for your own care. This does not mean that you are going to take over your own care. But it does mean that you should understand what is involved in your care.

- **You should talk with your doctor about your illness, and you should request written information or information about how to obtain written material.** Often your doctor will provide some background material spontaneously. However, people learn things in different ways, and what you receive may not be ideal for your particular needs. Here is a list of ways to get background information about your condition:

  - Talk with your doctor and/or the health-care team associated with your doctor. If your doctor seems unavailable, see if his or her staff can help you. If you are not satisfied with the explanations you receive, express this directly— politely, without anger, for the best results. Your doctor is likely very busy and may truly not be able to spend as much time with you as you'd like. But you can maximize the time you do spend together by preparing your questions in advance.

- Ask for written material about your health problem. Many doctors either write out explanations for their patients or have pamphlets and books about their particular health problems.
- Ask if there are videotapes explaining about the type of problem you have. Background information may be available via this route.
- Seek support groups that disseminate information.
- Call hot lines at your hospital or elsewhere in your area.
- Consult your local medical library.
- Read national journals such as *Science Week* that typically have sections on health-care breakthroughs.
- **Ask questions about changes in your therapy and about why certain steps are being taken.** It is likely that changes are non-negotiable. But how you feel about it may help your doctor make a decision about medication, about procedures, and about every aspect of your care. If your doctor doesn't know how you feel, then he or she may suggest a regimen that makes sense to him or her, but not to you.
- Prepare your questions. Jot your concerns and musings down as they occur to you. Get in the habit of doing this. Then:
  - Make a list of questions before your visit to the doctor. Make sure you bring the list.
  - If you find medically related articles in the newspaper or in magazines that you need explained or that lead you to question how your case is being handled, consider carrying them along to your visit. Show them to your doctor.
  - Keep notes about your physical state and any new symptoms you have. These do not need to be elaborate notes.

However, it can be invaluable to document what happens and when. For example, you could write:

7/1/96: Noticed white patches on my tongue after brushing my teeth. No fever, patches don't hurt.

This entry would mark that you had developed oral thrush. Your doctor could help by adding nystatin swish-and-swallow to your regimen to help you get rid of this. If you didn't note it, he or she might not know when this happened.

Do all doctors want to hear details from their patients and form an open interaction and partnership? Probably not. But with so much health-related information readily accessible, more and more patients are asking for this kind of relationship. Especially when their problems are chronic, ongoing ones.

My personal view is that, insofar as possible, there should be full disclosure by doctors and other health-care professionals. By this, I mean that both the doctor and the patient should share the relevant information about a given problem. This does not have to mean that every visit to your doctor's office will take an hour. It means that your doctor should aim to provide the background for your understanding about each problem. Obviously, a doctor cannot spend an hour discussing a pimple or poison ivy. But a doctor certainly can direct patients to the information and explanations appropriate to his or her medical background. A doctor should want to be a teacher as well as a healer.

Steroids: Types, Potency, Brands

In this section we have provided tables that note types of steroid preparations, their relative strengths (or potencies), and their brand names. However, we would like to point out that these lists are not exhaustive. We suggest that you talk with your health-care provider about your own medication program.

Steroid Drug Interactions

The following types of medicines can interact with steroids.

Class of Medication	Effect
Hepatic microsomal inducing drugs (barbituates, phenytoin, refampin)	Increase metabolism of glucocorticoids
Estrogens	Increase binding of steroids to transcortin
Nonsteroidal Anti-inflammatory Drugs:	
Indocin	Increase blood levels of steroids
Aspirin	Levels of aspirin increase when a person takes steroids
Potassium-Depleting Drugs: Diuretics may enhance the potassium-wasting effect of glucocorticoids	Increase renal loss of potassium
Anticholinesterase Agents. (ambenonium, neostigmine or pyridostigmine)	Given with steroids, cause weakness
Cyclosporine A	Decreased clearance of steroids
Oral Anticoagulants	Increased anticoagulant requirements

Adapted from: McEvoy JK, AHFS 96 American Society of Health-System Pharmacists, AHFS, 1996.

Types of Steroid Dosage

Term	Amount
Physiological or Replacement	The amount of glucocorticoid normally secreted by the adrenal cortex in a day (Usually 20 mg hydrocortisone, which is equal to 4 mg of prednisone/day)
Pharmacologic Doses	Any daily amount that is greater than a physiologic dose
Low Dose	A dosage slightly higher than physiologic (e.g., 5–15 mg prednisone daily)
Moderate dose	A dose of 0.5 mg of prednisone/kilogram of body weight each day
High dose	1–3 mg of prednisone/kilogram of body weight per day
Massive dose	15–30 mg of prednisone/kilogram each day

Adapted from: McEvoy JK, AHFS 96 American Society of Health-System Pharmacists, AHFS, 1996.

Equivalent Doses of Oral Steroids

Steroid Drug	Dosage Equivalent
Cortisone	25 mg
Hydrocortisone	20 mg
Prednisolone	5 mg
Prednisone	5 mg
Methylprednisone	4 mg
Methylprednisolone	4 mg
Triamcinolone	4 mg
Paramethasone Acetate	2 mg
Dexamethasone	0.750 mg
Betamethasone	0.6 mg

Note: The doses here are compared to cortisone. Thus, for example, prednisone is 5 times stronger, milligram for milligram than cortisone (25 milligrams of cortisone gives the same relative strength of 5 milligrams of prednisone. 25/5 = 5).

Source: McEvoy JK, AHFS 96 American Society of Health-System Pharmacists, AHFS, 1996, p2224.

Oral Corticosteroid Preparations

Generic Name (Chemical Name)	Brand Names	Pill Size or Syrup Strength	Special Comment
Beclomethasone (flubenisolone)	Celestone Celestone Syrup (has 1% alcohol and propylene glycol)	0.6 mg 0.6 mg/teaspoon (5 ml)	Minimal mineralocortoid effect; should not be used alone in patients with adrenal insufficiency
Cortisone Acetate (compound E)	Cortisone Acetate Tablets Cortone	5, 10 mg 25 mg	Drug of Choice for adrenal insufficiency; given several times per day
Dexamethasone (dexamethasone)	Decadron Tablets Decadron Elixir Dexamethasone Tablets Dexamethasone Intensol Solution Dexone Tablets	0.25, 0.5, 0.75, 1.5, 4, 6 mg 0.5 mg/teaspoon 1, 2 mg 0.5 mg/teaspoon 0.5, 0.75, 1.5, 4 mg	Used for anti-inflammatory or immunosuppression; used in endocrine testing; used in high doses to prevent vomiting in cancer chemotherapy
Fludrocortisone Acetate (fluohydrocortisone acetate fluohydrisone acetate 9α-fluorohydrocortisone acetate)	Florinef Acetate	0.1 mg	For adrenal insufficiency; for salt-losing forms of congenital adrenal hyperplasia; for treating postural low blood pressure (postural hypotension)
Hydrocortisone (compound F cortisol)	Cortef Hydrocortone	5, 10, 20 mg 10, 20 mg	Drug of choice for replacement therapy in adrenal insufficiency
Methylprednisolone (6-α-methylprednisolone)	Medrol Methylprednisolone Tablets	2,4,8,16, 24, 32 mg 16 mg	Used mainly as an anti-inflammatory and immunosuppressive; should not be used alone in in adrenal insufficiency

Oral Corticosteroid Preparations, *continued*

Paramethasone Acetate	Haldrone	2 mg	Used mainly as an anti-inflammatory/immuno-suppressive; don't use alone in adrenal insufficiency
Prednisolone	Cortalone	5 mg	Used mainly as an anti-inflammatory and immuno-suppressive; should not be used alone in adrenal insufficiency
	Delta-Cortef	5 mg	
	Prelone Syrup	15 mg/tsp (5 ml)	
Prednisone (deltacortisone deltahydrocortisone)	Deltasone	2.5, 5, 10, 20, 50 mg	Most commonly used glu-cocorticoid. Precautions as for prednisolone
	Orasone	1, 5, 10, 20, 50 mg	
	Meticorten	1 mg	
	Cortan	5, 20 mg	
	Panasol	5 mg	
	Steripred Unipack	5 mg	
	Steripred DS Unipak	10mg	
	Prednicen-M (coated)	5 mg	
	Prednisone Oral Sclution (with 5% alcohol)	5mg/tsp. (5ml)	
	Liquid Pred Syrup (with 5% alcohol)	5mg/tsp. (5ml)	
	Predisone Intensol (with 30% alcohol)	5 mg/ml	
Triamcinolone (triamcinolone)	Aristocort	1,2,4,8 mg	Most commonly used glu-cocorticoid. Precautions as for prednisolone
	Kenacort	4, 8 mg	
	Aristocort Syrup	2 mg/tsp. (5 ml)	
	Kenacort Diacetate Syrup	4 mg/tsp. (5 ml)	

Information taken from: McEvoy JK, AHFS 96 American Society of Health-System Pharmacists, AHFS, 1996.

Intravenous (IV) or Intramuscular (IM) Corticosteroids and Their Uses

Generic Name/(Chemical Name)	Brand Names	Uses
Betamethasone Sodium Phosphate Betamethasone Sodium Phosphate with Betamethasone Acetate	Celestone, Cel-U-Jec, Selestoject Celestone Soluspan	Can be given into joints, muscle and soft tissue, as well as intravenously. Anti-inflammatory and immunosuppressive; dose depends on condition.
Cortisone Acetate	Cortone Acetate	Intravenous or intramuscular adrenal replacement therapy; dose depends on condition. Relatively short-acting
Dexamethasone	IV or IM: Cortastat, Dalalone, Dexasone, Hexadrol Phosphate, Solurex, Dexacen IV only: Decadron Phosphate	Used IV for many emergencies: e.g., shock, cerebral edema, allergic conditions, severe asthma. Used as an IM injection for joint/muscle/or soft tissue inflammation.
Hydrocortisone	Hydrocortone, A-hydroCort, Solu-Cortef, Hydrocortisone Sodium Succinate	Same as for Cortisone Acetate Relatively short-acting
Methylprednisolone	IM: Depo-Medrol, Depoject, Depopred, Duralone, Medralone, Methylone, Rep-Pred IV: A-methaPred, Solu-Medrol Methylprednisolone Sodium Succinate	Injected into muscle, joints, tissue Relatively long-acting. Intravenous brands; longer-acting than hydrocortisone or cortisone. Used for many emergencies. Dose depends on condition.

Intravenous (IV) or Intramuscular (IM) Corticosteroids and Their Uses, *continued*

Prednisolone

Prednisolone Sodium Phosphate	Hydedeltrasol, Key-Pred, Nor-Pred; Predate S	Used IV or IM. Indications as for methylprednisolone
Prednisolone Tebutate	Hydeltra-T.B.A., Nor-Pred-T.B.A. Predalone T.B.A., Predate TBA, Predcor-TBA	Injected into muscle, joints, tissue Relatively long-acting

Triamcinolone

Triamcinolone Diacetate	Aristocort, Amcort, Articulose, Cenocort, Cinalone, Triam-Forte, Triamcinolone Forte, Tramolone 40, Trilone, Tristoject	Injected into muscle, joints, tissue
Triamcinolone Acetonide	Kenalong, Cenocort, Cinonide Kenaject, Kenalog, Tac-3 or -4, Triam-A, Triamonide, Tri-Kort, Trilog	Injected into muscle, joints, tissue
Triamcinolone Hexacetonide	Aristospan intralesional Aristospan Intra-articular	Injected into muscle, joints, tissue

Information taken from: McEvoy JK, AHFS 96 American Society of Health-System Pharmacists, AHFS, 1996.

Topical Corticosteroid Preparations

Topical steroids (placed on skin or on mucous membranes) can be used as local anti-inflammatory agents, most often in low dosage and only briefly. However, topical steroids can be prescribed as long-term treatment on the skin for conditions such as psoriasis, severe atopic dermatitis, or neurodermatitis. Steroids are also given as retention enemas in conditions such as ulcerative colitis and anorectal disorders (see chart of steroid preparations used in enema or suppository form).

Some of the lower-potency topical preparations are available over the counter. They should NEVER be used chronically without a doctor's guidance. In general, steroid creams, ointments and gels should not be used on the face, as these preparations may cause permanent skin changes. It must be remembered that topical steroids can be absorbed into the body and may, long-term, have generalized (systemic) effects and side effects.

You should be aware that the many topical steroids available have substantial differences in their inflammatory action. These preparations can be placed into relative potency groups (in decreasing order, with Group I being most potent). The following lists some of these preparations:

Generic Names	Trade Names
Group I	
Betamethasone dipropionate cream	Diprolene
Clobetasol propionate cream or ointment	Temovate
Diflorasone diacetate ointment	Psorcon
Group II	
Amcinonide ointment	Cyclocort
Betamethasone dipropionate ointment	Diprosone
Desoximetasone cream or ointment	Topicort
Desoximetasone gel	Topicort
Diflorasone diacetate ointment	Florone, Maxiflor
Fluocinonide cream or ointment	Lidex
Fluocinonide gel	—
Halcinonide cream	Halog

Generic Names	*Trade Names*

Group III

Betamethasone benzoate gel	
Betamethasone dipropionate cream	Diprosone
Betamethasone valerate ointment	Valisone
Diflorasone diacetate cream	Florone, Maxiflor
Mometasone furoate ointment	Elocon
Triamcinolone acetonide cream	Aristocort

Group IV

Desoximetasone cream	Topicort
Fluocinolone acetonide cream	Synalar-HP
Fluocinolone acetonide ointment	Synalar
Flurandrenolide ointment	Cordran
Triamcinolone acetonide ointment	Aristocort, Kenalog

Group V

Betamethasone benzoate cream	—
Betamethasone dipropionate lotion	Diprosone
Betamethasone valerate cream or lotion	Valisone
Fluocinolone acetonide cream	Synalar
Flurandrenolide cream	Cordran
Hydrocortisone butyrate cream	Locoid
Hydrocortisone valerate cream	Westcort
Prednicarbate cream	Dermatop Emollient
Triamcinolone acetonide cream or lotion	Kenalog

Group VI

Alclometasone dipropionate cream or oint.	Aclovate
Desonide cream	Tridesilon
Fluocinolone acetonide solution	Synalar

Information taken from: McEvoy JK, AHFS 96 American Society of Health-System Pharmacists, AHFS, 1996.

Steroid Preparations Used in Enema or Suppository Form

Generic	Trade Name	Comment
Hydrocortisone	Cortenema	Single dose retention enema (100 mg per enema)
	Proctocort	Cream
	Anucort-HC	Suppository
	Anusol-HC	
	Cort-Dome High Potency	
	Hemorrhoidal-HC	
	Hemril-HC Uniserts	
Hydrocortisone Acetate	Cortifoam	Rectal foam (80 mg of hydrocortisone/dose)
	Proctofoam HC	

Information taken from: McEvoy JK, AHFS 96 American Society of Health-System Pharmacists, AHFS, 1996.

Inhaled/Intranasal Corticosteroid Preparations

Generic Name (Chemical Name)	Brand Names	Dosage Information	Special Comment
Beclomethasone Dipropionate	Beclovent Oral Inhaler Vanceril Oral Inhaler	42 µg/metered spray	Used in asthma
	Beconase Inhalation Aerosol Vancenase Nasal Inhaler	42 µg/metered spray	Used intranasally
	Beconase AQ Nasal Spray Vancenase AQ Nasal Spray	Equivalent to 42 micrograms	
Budesonide	Rhinocort	50µg/metered spray	Used intranasally
Dexamethasone Sodium Phosphate	Decadron Phosphate Respihaler Dexacort Phosphate Respihaler	100 µg/metered spray	Used in asthma and bronchospasm
Flunisolide	AeroBid Inhaler System Aerobid-M	250 µg/metered spray	Used in asthma and bronchospasm
	Nasalide 0.025%	25 µg/metered spray	Used for rhinitis, allergies, eustachian tube swelling
Fluticasone Propionate	Flonase Nasal Spray	50 µg/metered spray	Used for rhinitis, allergies, eustachian tube swelling
Triamcinolone Acetonide	Asthmacort Oral Inhaler	100 µg/metered spray	Used in asthma

Note: µg = microgram

Information taken from: McEvoy JK, AHFS 96 American Society of Health-System Pharmacists, AHFS, 1996.

Ophthalmic (Eye) Corticosteroid Preparations

Comment: Steroids come as sterile solutions, suspensions or ointments for use in the eyes. Ointments stay in the eye longest but interfere with vision, so are usually used at night, or to treat problems with the eyelids, while solutions or suspensions are used during the day. Steroids are often combined with anti-infective therapy to treat bacterial infection. Corticosteroids given alone are generally contraindicated in herpetic infection of the eye, although a combination of anti-viral agent with steroids has been used with some success.

Generic Name (Chemical Name)	Brand Names
Dexamethasone	Suspension: Maxidex (0.1%)
Dexamethasone (0.1%) with Neomycin and Polymyxin B	Ointments: AK-Trol, Dexacidin, Dexasporin, Maxitrol, Ocu-Trol Suspension: AK-Trol, Dexacidin, Dexasporin, Dex-ide, Maxitrol Ocu-Trol
Dexamethasone (0.1%) with Tobramycin	Ointment: TobraDex Suspension: TobraDex
Dexamethasone Sodium Phosphate with Neomycin Sulfate	Ointment: NeoDecadron Solution: AK-Neo-Dex
Fluorometholone	Ointment: FML S.O.P. (0.1%) Suspension: Fluor-Op (0.1%), FML Liquifilm (0.1%), FML Forte Liquifilm (0.25%)
Fluorometholone with Sulfacetamide	Suspension: FML-S Liquifilm
Fluorometholone Acetate	Flarex (0.1%)
Hydrocortisone with Neomycin Polymyxin B Sulfate, Bacitracin Zinc	Ointment: AK Spore HC, Cortisporin Ophthalmic

Ophthalmic (Eye) Corticosteroid Preparations, *continued*

Hydrocortisone with Neomycin and Polymyxin B Sulfate	Suspension: AK-Spore Suspension, Cortisporin Ophthalmic Suspension
Hydrocortisone Acetate with Chloramphenicol and Polymyxin B Sulfate	Ophthocort
Hydrocortisone Acetate with Neomycin, Polymyxin B Sulfate, Bacitracin Zinc	Ointment: Neotricin HC
Hydrocortisone Acetate with Oxytetracycline	Suspension: Terra-Cortril
Prednisolone Acetate	Suspension: Pred Mild (0.12%), Econopred (0.125%), EconopredPlus (1%), PredForte (1%)
Prenisolone Acetate and Gentamicin	Ointment: Pred-G S.O.P. Suspension: Pred-G Liquifilm
Prednisolone Acetate and Neomycin and Polymyxin B Sulfates	Suspension: Poly-Pred Liquifilm
Prednisolone Acetate and Sulfacetamide	Ointment: Blephamide, Cetapred AK-Cide, Metimyd, Vasocidin
	Suspension: Blephamide Liquifilm, Isoptocetapred, AK-Cide, Metimyd
Prednisolone Sodium Phosphate	Solution: AK-Pred (0.125% or 1%), Inflamase Mild (0.125%), Inflamase Forte (1%)
Prednisolone Sodium Phosphate with Sulfacetamide Sodium	Solution: Sulster, Vasocidin

Information taken from: McEvoy JK, AHFS 96 American Society of Health-System Pharmacists, AHFS, 1996.

Optic (Ear) Corticosteroid Preparations

Comment: Steroids can be applied to the ear canal for the relief of inflammation there. It is important that any infection be eliminated or controlled before using steroids in the ear canal, unless appropriate antibiotics are used concomitantly. Sometimes steroids are used for chronic inflammation of the external ear canal, as may be seen in psoriasis, seborrhea, allergic dermatitis or neurodermatitis.

Generic Name	Brand Names
Hydrocortisone (1%) and Acetic Acid (2%)	Solution: Acetasol HC VoSol HC Otic Solution
Hydrocortisone and Neomycin Polymyxin B Sulfate	Solution: AK-Spore HC Otic Solution, Antibiotic Ear Solution, Cortatrigen Otic Solution, Cortisporin Otic Solution, Drotic Ear Drops, LazerSporin-C, Otocort Ear Solution
	Suspension: AK-Spore HC Otic Suspension, Antibiotic Ear Suspension, Cortatrigen Otic Suspension, Otocort Ear Suspension, PediOtic Suspension, UAD Otic Suspension
Hydrocortisone and Polymyxin B Sulfate	Otobiotic
Hydrocortisone Acetate and Neomycin and Colistin Sulfate	Coly-Mycin S Otic with Neomycin and Hydrocortisone

Information taken from: McEvoy JK, AHFS 96 American Society of Health-System Pharmacists, AHFS, 1996.

NEW Steroid Preparations Soon to be Generally Available

Budesonide

Budesonide is the generic name of a new steroid medication that is very potent and holds great promise for treatment of asthma, nasal polyps, and gastrointestinal conditions. It has been used in Europe for some time, both as an inhalant or nasal preparation, and in rectal preparations. The drug can also be administered orally. A nasal preparation (Rhinocort) has been approved by the Food and Drug Administration in the United States. Other preparations are being evaluated.

Other Steroids

In the next months and years, additional formulations of steroids will become available. As an informed patient, you should be vigilant in seeking the latest about new medications.

In the future, steroid preparations that are inhaled or sprayed will be free of propellants that pose any problem to the environment. Name brands may change as a result.

The diagram on the following page depicts the interrelationships of various steroid compounds synthesized by the adrenal glands. All originate from cholesterol. The synthesis of aldosterone (and other so-called mineralocorticoids) and the synthesis of cortisol (and other so-called glucocorticoids) are placed to the left of the vertical line. The synthesis of sex hormones is shown to the right of the vertical line. The dashed rectangles contain the names of enzymes that do the chemical work to produce one form of steroid from another.

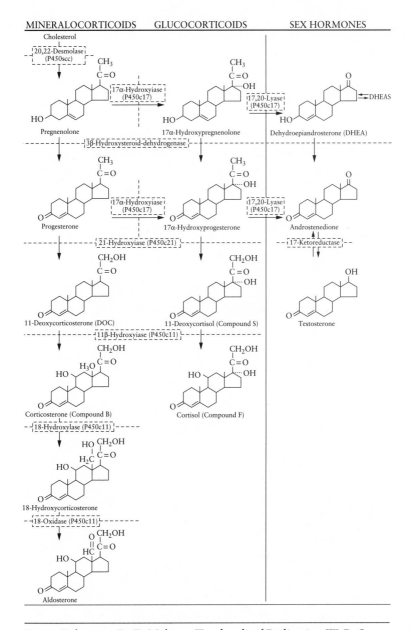

From: Behrman, R. E. Nelson, *Textbook of Pediatrics,* W. B. Saunders Company, Philadelphia, PA, 1992, p. 1442.

AIDS

AIDS Clinical Trials
   Information Service
PO Box 6421
Rockville, MD 20849-6421
PHONE: 800-TRIALS-A
            (874-2572)
            800-243-7012
            (TTD deficiency access line)
FAX: 301-738-6616
E-MAIL: actis@cdcnac.org
*NOTE: Calls to NIH or to the
CDC (see above) will get you
into the vast AIDS-related
information networks.*

Cancer Treatment

ACS
American Cancer Society
1599 Clifton Road, NE
Atlanta, GA 30329
PHONE: 800-227-2345
            (ACS-2345)
            (National Office)
            404-320-3333
FAX: 404-329-5787

Cancer Information Service
1-800-4-CANCER

National Cancer Institute
Office of Communications
NIH
9000 Rockville Pike
Building 31, Room 10A31
Bethesda, MD 20892
PHONE: 301-496-6631
FAX: 301-402-4945
E-MAIL: occ.nci.nih.gov

Dermatologic Problems

American Academy of
   Dermatology
930 North Meacham Road
Schaumberg, IL 60173-4965
PHONE: 847-330-0230
FAX: 847-330-0050
WWW SITE:
            http://www/aad.org

American Skin Association
150 East 5th Street, 58th Street,
   33rd Floor
New York, NY 10155-0002
PHONE: 212-753-8260
FAX: 212-688-6547

Dermatology Foundation
1560 Sherman Avenue
Evanston, IL 60201-4802
PHONE: 847-328-2256
FAX: 847-328-0509
EMAIL: dfgen@dermfnd.org

Eczema Association for Science
and Education
1221 SW Yamhill, Suite 303
Portland, OR 97205
PHONE: 503-228-4430
FAX: 503-273-8778

National Psoriasis Foundation
6600 SW 92d Street, Suite 300
Portland, OR 97223
PHONE: 800-723-9166
              503-244-7404
FAX: 503-245-0626

Endocrine Problems

Cushing's Support and Research
Foundation
65 East India Row, 22B
Boston, MA 02110
PHONE: 617-723-3674

The Endocrine Society
4350 East West Highway
Suite 500
Bethesda, MD 20814-4410
PHONE: 301-941-0252
Physician Referral Line:
              1-800-HORMONE
FAX: 301-941-0259
E-MAIL:
              endostaff@endo-society.org

NADF (National Adrenal
Diseases Foundation)
505 Northern Boulevard
Great Neck, NY 11021
PHONE: 516-487-4992
EMAIL: nads@aol.com
WWW SITE:
              http://medhlp.netusa.net/
              www/nadf.htm

Thyroid Foundation of
America, Inc.
Ruth Sleeper Hall, RSL 350
40 Parkman Street
Boston, MA 02114
PHONE: 800-832-8321
FAX: 617-726-4136
WWWSITE:
              TFAweb.org/pob/tfa

Eye Problems

American Academy of
Ophthalmology
PO Box 7424
San Francisco, CA 94120-7424
PHONE: 415-561-8500
FAX: 415-561-8533
WWWSITE:
              http://www.eyenet.org

National Eye Research
Foundation
910 Skokie Boulevard, #207A
Northbrook, IL 60062
PHONE: 800-621-2258
              847-564-4652
FAX: 847-564-0807

Gastrointestinal Problems

American Dietetic Association
216 West Jackson Boulevard
Chicago, IL 60606
PHONE: 312-899-0040
FAX: 312-899-4845
              (Public Relations FAX)

American Liver Foundation
1425 Pompton Avenue
Cedar Grove, NJ 07009
PHONE: 800-223-0179
        201-256-2550
FAX: 201-256-3214
WWWSITE:
http://www.LiverFoundation.org

Crohn's and Colitis Foundation
    of America, Inc.
3286 Park Avenue South, 17th
    Floor
New York, NY 10016-8804
PHONE: 800-932-2423
        212-685-3440
FAX: 212-779-4098

Digestive Disease National
    Coalition
507 Capital Court Suite 200
Washington, DC 20002
PHONE: 202-544-7497
FAX: 202-546-7105

National Digestive Diseases
    Information Clearinghouse
2 Information Way
Bethesda, MD 20892-3570
PHONE: 301-654-3810
FAX: 301-907-8906
www: http://www.nih.gov.
        or
        http://www.niddk.gov

Hearing Problems

Deafness Research Foundation
15 West 39th Street
New York, NY 10018
PHONE: 800-535-3323
        212-768-1181
FAX: 212-768-1782
E-MAIL: drf1.villageiof.com
WWWSITE:
        http://villageiof.comdrf1

Heart Problems

American Heart Association
7272 Greenville Avenue
Dallas, TX 75231-4596
PHONE: 800-242-8721
        214-373-6300
FAX: 214-369-3685

Kidney Problems

AAKP (American Association of
    Kidney Patients)
100 S. Ashley Drive, Suite 280
Tampa, FL 33602
PHONE: 800-749-2257
FAX: 813-223-0001
E-MAIL: AAKPnat@aol.com

AKF (American Kidney Fund)
6110 Executive Boulevard,
    Suite 1010
Rockville, MD 20852
PHONE: 800-638-8299
        800-492-8361
        301-881-3052
FAX: 301-881-0898
E-MAIL: helpline@akfine.org
WWWSITE:
        http://www.arbon.com/kidney

NKF (National Kidney
   Foundation)
30 East 33d Street
New York, NY 10016
PHONE: 800-622-9010
          212-889-2210
FAX: 212-689-9261
WWW SITE:
       http://www.kidney.org

Lung (Pulmonary) Problems

American Lung Association
1740 Broadway
New York, NY 10019-4374
PHONE: 800-LUNG-USA
          212-315-8700
FAX: 212-265-5642
          212-315-8872
          (communication)

Asthma and Allergy Foundation
   of America
1125 15th Street, NW, Suite 502
Washington, DC 20005
PHONE: 800-7-ASTHMA
          202-466-7643
          (National Office)

Neurological Problems

Multiple Sclerosis Foundation
6350 North Andrews Avenue
Fort Lauderdale, FL 33309
PHONE: 800-441-7055
          954-776-6805
FAX: 954-938-8708
E-MAIL: msfacts@icanect.net

Rheumatology/ Autoimmune Diseases

Arthritis Foundation
National Office
1330 West Peachtree Street
Atlanta, GA 30309
PHONE: 800-283-7800

Lupus Foundation of America
1300 Piccard Drive, Suite 200
Rockville, MD 20850-4303
PHONE: 800-558-0121
          301-670-9292
FAX: 301-670-9486
WWWSITE:
       http://www.lupus.org/lupus

Selected References about Glucocorticoids

NOTE: *These few articles chosen from among thousands contain jump-off points for the reader who wishes to go further. Many of these articles are technical and may require some "translating" if you do not have a science background. Annotations are included beneath citations as indicated. The articles are in chronological order.*

Medical Articles

Hench, P. S., E. C. Kendall, C. H. Slocumb, and H. F. Polley. The effect of a hormone of the adrenal cortex (17-Hydroxy-11-dehydro-corticosterone: Compound E) and of pituitary adrenocorticotropic hormone on rheumatoid arthritis; preliminary report. *Proceedings of Staff Meetings of the Mayo Clinic* 24: 181–97, 1949.
  Pathfinding first article by Dr. Hench, who later won the Nobel Prize for his and his group's work.

Hench, P. S. The reversibility of certain rheumatic and nonrheumatic conditions, by the use of cortisone or of the pituitary adrenocorticotropic hormone. *Annals of Internal Medicine* 36: 1–38, 1952.
  Important article by Nobelist P. Hench.

Rome, H., and F. Braceland. The psychological response to ACTH, cortisone, hydrocortisone and related steroid substances. *American Journal of Psychiatry* 108: 641–51, 1952.
  Early study about psychological responses to ACTH and glucocorticoids.

Axelrod, L. Glucocorticoid therapy. *Medicine* (Baltimore) 55: 39–65, 1976.
  Good early review about therapy and side effects.

Ling, M. H., F. J. Perry, and M. T. Tsuang. Side effects of corticosteroid therapy. Psychiatric aspects. *Archives of General Psychiatry* 38: 471–77, 1981.

Baylink, D. J. Glucocorticoid-induced osteoporosis. *New England Journal of Medicine* 309: 306–08, 1983.
   Steroids and bone problems.

Lewis, D. A., and P. E. Smith. Steroid induced psychiatric syndromes. A report of 14 cases and a review of the literature. *Journal of Affective Disorders* 5: 319–32, 1983.

Lucky, A. W. Principles of the use of glucocorticosteroids in the growing child. *Pediatric Dermatology* 1: 226–35, 1984.
   Article on use of glucocorticoids in children.

Schleimer, R. P., H. N. Claman, and A. L. Oronsky (eds.). *Antiinflammatory Steroid Action: Basic and Clinical Aspects.* Academic Press, Inc., NY, 1989, 564 pp.
   Excellent text with much background on how steroids work and their side effects. Many contributors.

Wolkowitz, O. M., D. Rubinow, A. A. Doran, et al. Prednisone effects on neurochemistry and behavior. Preliminary findings. *Archives of General Psychiatry* 47: 963–68, 1990.

Reckart, M. D., and S. J. Eisendrath. Exogenous corticosteroid effects on mood and cognition: Case presentations. *International Journal of Psychosomatic Diseases* 37: 57–61, 1990.

Satel, S. L. Mental status changes in children receiving glucocorticoids. Review of the literature. *Clinical Pediatrics* 29: 383–88, 1990.

Klein, J. F. Adverse psychiatric effects of systemic glucocorticoid therapy. *American Family Physician* 46: 1469–74, 1992.

Salem, M., R. E. Tainish, Jr., J. Bromberg, D. L. Loriaux, and B. Chernow. Perioperative glucocorticoid coverage. A reassessment 42 years after emergence of a problem. *Annals of Surgery* 219: 416–25, 1994.
   Information about how to manage patients who have been on steroids and need an operation.

Barnes, P. J. Inhaled glucocorticoids for asthma. *New England Journal of Medicine* 332: 868–75, 1995.
   Review about inhaled steroids in reactive airway disease.

Cato, A. C., Wade E. Molecular mechanisms of anti-inflammatory action of glucocorticoids. *Bioessays* 18: 371–78, 1996.

Up-to-date review of how steroids carry out their anti-inflammatory actions.

Essays/Films

Roueché, Berton. "Ten Feet Tall." *New Yorker,* 1955. (September 10, p 47)

Bigger Than Life, film starring James Mason, 1956, director Nicholas Ray.
The compelling drama of teacher Mason, who becomes hooked on cortisone, and its devastating effects on him and his family.

INDEX